BIRTH CRISIS

When a woman is denied all choice – feels as if she has been swallowed up by a vast machine and spat out at the other end with a baby – how can she move on from there?

We probably all know someone who is distressed after childbirth. She has been told to pull herself together, be grateful for her beautiful baby, and is likely to have been prescribed anti-depressants. She may conceal her pain, but it can fester for years. In *Birth Crisis* Sheila Kitzinger explores women's experiences and their resulting anxiety. Topics include:

* increasing intervention in pregnancy
* the emphasis on technological surveillance
* how family, friends and caregivers can respond to the needs of trau-matized mothers
* why those working in the maternity system should promote change.

Birth Crisis draws on the thousands of hours Sheila has listened to women's wide-ranging experiences and her knowledge of the maternity system.

She reveals the causes of this suffering, which has, until now, been brushed under the carpet. Her book is an essential resource for student and practising midwives and health professionals, as well as women and those close to them who want to learn how to come to terms with and heal the trauma.

Sheila Kitzinger is one of the leading authorities on childbirth. She has been described as 'the high priestess' of the birth movement and lectures in many countries. She is a vigorous campaigner for the rights of women in matters of birth, motherhood and sex and is a widely published author. Her books include *Understanding Your Crying Baby*, *The Politics of Birth*, *The New Experience of Childbirth*, *The New Pregnancy and Childbirth*, *Birth Your Way*, *Rediscovering Birth* and *Talking with Children about Things that Matter*.

BIRTH CRISIS

SHEILA KITZINGER

Routledge
Taylor & Francis Group

LONDON AND NEW YORK

First published 2006 by Routledge
2 Park Square, Milton Park, Abingdon, Oxon OX14 4RN

Simultaneously published in the USA and Canada
by Routledge
270 Madison Avenue, New York, NY 10016

Reprinted 2007

Routledge is an imprint of the Taylor & Francis Group, an informa business

Typeset in Times by
Florence Production Ltd, Stoodleigh, Devon
Printed and bound in Great Britain by
TJ International Ltd, Padstow, Cornwall

British Library Cataloguing in Publication Data
A catalogue record for this book is available from
the British Library

Library of Congress Cataloging in Publication Data
Kitzinger, Sheila.
 Birth crisis/Sheila Kitzinger.
  p. cm.
 Includes bibliographical references and index.
   1. Childbirth – Psychological aspects.   2. Labor (Obstetrics) –
Psychological aspects.   3. Delivery (Obstetrics) – Psychological aspects.
4. Post-traumatic stress disorder.   5. Psychic trauma.   6. Mothers –
Mental health.   I. Title.
 RG658.K566 2006
 618.4 – dc22   2005034724

ISBN10: 0–415–37265–8 (hbk)
ISBN10: 0–415–37266–6 (pbk)
ISBN10: 0–203–96872–7 (ebk)

ISBN13: 978–0–415–37265–7 (hbk)
ISBN13: 978–0–415–37266–4 (pbk)

CONTENTS

vii

ACKNOWLEDGEMENTS

SPECIAL THANKS TO my daughter Tess McKenney for all her research and computer skills, together with her wisdom and common sense. The distinctive look of this book is thanks to Jo Nesbitt's witty cover illustration. My warm thanks also to the women who have shared with me their birth stories and their often intense and disturbing emotions. The drawings they have sent me vividly convey the images of their nightmares and flashbacks. I am grateful to Erin Horsley for her dramatic drawings in Chapters 3 and 6, and Uwe Kitzinger for the photographs in Chapters 2 and 8. With many thanks to Deirdrie Cullen the photographer, and the women who posed for her, for the eight gorgeous photographs in the other chapters of this book. They did this, with great generosity, to promote the Maternity Coalition, to publicise the reforms that need to be made in maternity care in Australia, and to promote one-to-one midwifery and choices in Australia.

The chapter on sexual abuse and birth owes a great deal to research that my daughter Professor Jenny Kitzinger has done. I want to thank my colleague in Seattle, Penny Simkin, too, for her major contribution to understanding distress in childbirth following sexual abuse. The book she wrote with Phyllis Klaus will become a classic. I am grateful to research midwife and lecturer Ethel Burns for help with the code to case notes in Chapter 12. I'd like to thank my colleagues in the National Childbirth Trust and the Association for Improvements in the Maternity Services for all the positive work they do to help women.

Robbie Davis-Floyd's sociological analysis of maternity care and midwifery is a spur to critical thinking and an understanding of power politics in the health services.

I am also grateful to those women who agreed that I could tape our discussions on the phone for transcribing and using as vivid material for conversation analysis undertaken by my daughter Professor Celia Kitzinger. The conversations presented in dramatic form (as if they were from the script of a play) are selected from the data of over 560 tapes.

Emmeline Crause, my assistant, has worked with commitment to make this book a reality, and is very good at multi-tasking. She's off to a great future in Australia.

ACKNOWLEDGEMENTS

ABBREVIATIONS

AIMS	Association for Improvements in the Maternity Services
ARM	artificial rupture of membranes
CTG	cardiotocograph
EDD	expected date of delivery
EFM	electronic fetal monitoring
GP	General Practitioner
HBAC	home birth after Caesarean
IMA	Independent Midwives Association
LMP	last menstrual period
MIDIRS	Midwife's Information and Resource Service
NCT	National Childbirth Trust
NHS	National Health Service
PTSD	post-traumatic stress disorder
PUPPS	pruritic urticarial papules and plaques of pregnancy
RCOG	Royal College of Obstetricians and Gynaecologists
TENS	Transcutaneous Electronic Nerve Stimulation
VBAC	vaginal birth after Caesarean
WHO	World Health Organization

BIRTH 16 IX 78

The pod of my flesh
bulged and split
unwilling
to shed its fruit.
The doctor yelled
get out at my lover
and my friend who
held my hand.
I wanted her
to be kind.
Catheters were
inserted and
a rubber mask
went over my face.
They pierced my waters
with a pin.
We waited.
I watched for dawn.
Only waiting
in bright light,
the clink of trolleys
and smell
of germicide.
He was born
oh yes
as I lay draped
in a green gown
feet in the air
feeling nothing,

he was born.

I'm crying now
for that pain.
Scarred, I will
Never heal:
The skin on my belly
wrinkled with sudden age
my vulva stitched and raw
tits swollen and dripping.
Scared of dying.
He lay in a metal cot
with a tube in his nose
and his father cried.
I shall go on crying
until this birth is expiated.

The child sucks at me
Unerringly, without
gratitude.

I shall go on crying
until this birth
is expiated.

Lesley Saunders[1]

1 L. Saunders, 'Birth 16 ix 78', in R. Palmeira (ed.), *In the Gold of Flesh: Poems of Birth and Motherhood*, London, The Women's Press, 1990.

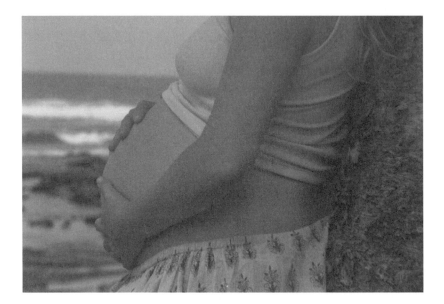

BIRTH SHOCK

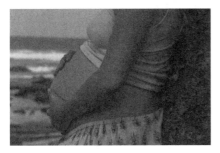

I LOOKED FORWARD to childbirth and though I felt a kind of stage fright before the first birth, I was never really anxious. I enjoyed giving birth. But then, all my babies were born at home, and I had one-to-one midwife care.

For many women it isn't like that. Research shows that one in every twenty new mothers is diagnosed with traumatic stress after childbirth.[1,2] Many others suffer but feel that doctors won't be able to help them, so they either don't tell their General Practitioner (GP), or seek help from a doctor but never get any medical diagnosis, or are mistakenly diagnosed as clinically depressed. Immediately after birth they are stunned, relieved that their ordeal is over. They may even be euphoric and thank the obstetrician who, they are told, rescued the baby from disaster. But after a few weeks or months this is followed by inner turmoil, with flashbacks, nightmares and panic attacks.

Many women avoid getting pregnant again because they can't face going through the same ordeal. Then panic subsides with time, and they think they have come to terms with the experience. They start another pregnancy, and after a few months it all comes rushing back and they are in a state of terror.

The next birth may be only weeks away. Why is birth traumatic? It is not only a matter of pain. Women are traumatised by being treated like machines that are at constant risk of breaking down. They are traumatised by feeling that they are sucked into a medical system that deprives them of any control over what is happening to them.

In northern industrial countries – and increasingly all over the world – our culture of birth is heavily medicalised. On TV, birth is presented as a medical event that is safe only in the hands of doctors, and if women obey the doctors, everything turns out all right. Those who ask questions or opt for home birth are setting themselves up for a medical emergency.

We also have to deal with a stereotyped and romanticised image of new motherhood. Think of the photographs of shining, starry-eyed women cradling their beautiful (usually sleeping) babies. How many of us really feel like that? And even if there are wonderful moments, what about the times in between? A woman who is distressed often thinks she must keep it a dark secret. No one wants to hear about her feelings of panic and failure. She believes she is different from all other mothers. They are coping. She is not. Look at the photographs of pop stars and 'celebs' who zip into shape and glisten with success within weeks of having an elective Caesarean. Why can't she be like them? What is wrong with her?

If she goes to her doctor, she may be told she is depressed and prescribed anti-depressants. But this is different from depression. Someone who is depressed wakes in the morning feeling unable to face the day. There is a terrible lethargy. Yet this woman is tense and anxious – constantly on 'red alert'. She is suffering from post-traumatic stress.

In the First World War the diagnosis was 'shell shock'. Veterans of the Vietnam War were first diagnosed as having post-traumatic stress disorder (PTSD) after being in situations where they were helpless and trapped. They had no physical injuries, but they were emotionally damaged. Soldiers on both sides of the conflict went through this, as have many others in wars since then. It can be the same for women after childbirth. It is a normal reaction to insensitive care when a woman has no choices and no means of escape.

In professional journals – psychiatric, medical, midwifery, for example – distress after birth is often discussed as a disease that strikes women who are especially vulnerable because of a pre-existing mental state. Their unhappiness has psychiatric labels stuck on it, and suffering is medically framed and individualised as an illness to be treated without any reference to the social context in which it occurs. One psychiatrist has pointed out that:

> *Any psychiatric diagnosis is primarily a way of seeing, a style of reasoning, and (in compensation suits or other claims) a means of persuasion . . . The medicalisation of life . . . tends to mean that distress is relocated from the social arena to the clinical arena.*[3]

When this happens, the way women are treated in childbirth, the failure of the maternity services to give humane care, can be ignored.

I have heard from so many women going through emotional trauma after birth that I set up and run a Birth Crisis Network, a phone line for women who need to talk about their fear of birth and their experiences of unhappy birth. I have learned that the important thing is to listen rather than give advice. This enables them gradually to find the power within themselves to deal with the trauma. They may say, 'You are the first person I have told.'

As we have seen, a GP may dismiss their distress as so common that it must be normal:

> *My GP said, 'What you are describing is quite normal. Be glad your baby's OK. Don't worry about it, dear.' So I asked to see the consultant and I complained about my treatment. He was very patronising and only got in touch with my GP, who told me I had post-natal depression and sent me to a psychologist. When she heard all about it, she said, 'You are justifiably angry.' I asked my GP for a second opinion. He said, 'What do you expect to gain from that? Don't be silly!' I feel I have been cheated of a normal birth, and they have all hidden things from me and deceived me.*

Women have often said they have tried to talk to their partners, family and friends, who have switched off because they have felt unable to help and are tired of hearing about it: 'You are not on about that again, are you?', 'Be thankful you have got a healthy baby', 'You expected too much', 'You were unrealistic about the birth', 'Put it behind you! Get on with your life!' But they can't. The events of the birth go round and round in their minds like a video that cannot be switched off.

Panic overwhelms them when they happen to see a pregnant woman, when they switch on a TV programme in which there is a birth or when they drive past the hospital. They withdraw into themselves, feeling stigmatised, turned into outcasts by their experience. A woman whose child is now two years old says, 'Everyone thinks I should be over it by now. I ask myself, "What is wrong with me? Why can't I cope like other women?"' They have sudden panic attacks and this, together with an intense sense of isolation, may make them feel they are going mad.

HOW IS BIRTH TURNED INTO AN ORDEAL?

Women in childbirth are treated like products on a factory conveyor belt. Technocracy distorts the birth experience. Their labours are obstetrically 'managed', and they feel they are not cared for as human beings, but are like 'meat on a table', 'an oven-trussed turkey' or 'fish on a slab'. They suffer from institutionalised violence. This has far-reaching consequences. It is likely to affect the way a woman feels not only about herself but also about her baby and her partner. It may have catastrophic effects on relationships.

A woman gave birth in a hospital where she was required to lie in a supine position throughout labour, had to deliver with her legs in stirrups, and had a large episiotomy that was badly sutured. She needed surgery to repair her perineum, and is still in pain months after. She is being advised to opt for a Caesarean with the next birth. But she says:

> I will never have any more children. I will not subject myself to that again. . . . I remember exactly what was done and said and by whom. I have the relentless torture of re-living this experience daily, especially at night. . . . The videotape is always going on in my head.

She went on to say: 'This experience has so traumatised me that I did not even speak about it for six months. I knew that it was totally out of character for me to bottle things up or deny that something was very wrong.'

This videotape image recurs again and again in women's accounts. Professor Cheryl Beck lists it as a major theme in PTSD and quotes a woman who said:

I lived in two worlds, the videotape of the birth and the 'real' world. The videotape felt more real. I lived in my own bubble, not quite connecting with anyone. I could hear and communicate, but experienced interaction with others as a spectator. The 'videotape' ran constantly for 4 months.

Another woman had a labour in which she said, 'I was just a case to them. They didn't speak *to* me, only *about* me.' That labour ended in a Caesarean section. Afterwards she told me:

My baby was next to me but I didn't want to touch him or look at him. I was mourning the loss of a child who never came through me. I was unable to give birth. He was stripped from me. Eight hours after the operation, the nurse came and asked me if I had touched my son and I said 'No.' She was worried that he hadn't had any milk and she put him straight away onto my breast which I found a bit of a shock. It was like meeting a man for the first time and even when you do not fancy him people make you kiss him on the lips.

In the UK over a third of women have an operative delivery, and most of these have epidural anaesthesia. They may not know why this has happened and feel that they have failed to achieve a normal birth.[4] Almost one woman in every four has a Caesarean. There is a 21 per cent induction rate, and 11 per cent of deliveries are instrumental. These high rates of obstetric intervention often make women feel helpless and disempowered. But it does not follow automatically that a woman who has an intervention will be distressed after birth. The quality of relationships with her caregivers is what matters most. When that is poor, even an apparently straightforward labour and a normal vaginal delivery can be traumatic. One woman said:

No one believes me. My GP thinks I am neurotic. She says, 'That's what happens when you have a baby. Millions of women all over the world have babies.' And I know what she means is 'And don't make this fuss.' Sometimes I feel I must be going out of my mind.

This book explores the way in which childbirth is managed in the twenty-first century, and the effect it has on women, couples and families. I look at how care needs to be changed, suggest ways in which post-traumatic stress after birth can be prevented and, when it does occur, how it can be healed.

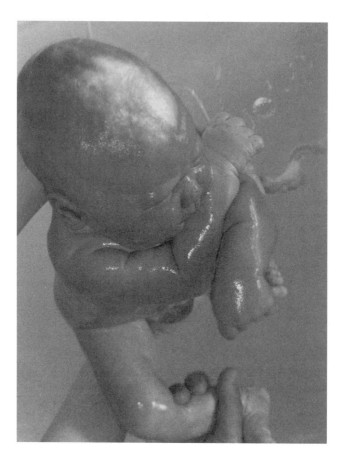

BIRTH CONTRASTS

2

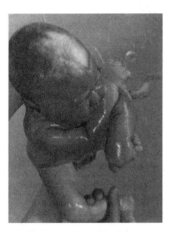

Two women discuss their births. For one it was among the happiest experiences of her life. The other looks back on it with horror, haunted by images of being trapped, helpless and in pain. She says that anyone who talks about birth as if it could be enjoyed must be either a masochist or a liar. She feels the ordeal endured is trivialised and dismissed by the woman who puts on an act of being radiant and triumphant. The two are unable to communicate other than through claim and counter-claim.

Birth experiences are often in such startling contrast that women learn not to talk about them, or make seemingly casual, throwaway comments in case they trigger hostility. One woman feels personally blamed for having a traumatic birth. Another feels accused of romanticising the reality in order to assert a kind of female superiority. For each of them the narrative they offer is real. For each the birth story becomes part of their lives and an important element in their identity.

The woman for whom birth was deeply satisfying was in an environment that she could control herself – not just the room and things in it but the people caring for her – and she laboured without interference. The one whose birth was distressing was denied all control, and was subjected to many interventions that started as induction or acceleration of labour and led to what was virtually a landslide of other interventions. Just as a landslide begins when one stone is dislodged and hits another, and then the second one begins rolling, and a third, until the earth disintegrates and crashes down the mountainside, so a medical act such as induction, or harpooning a woman to an electronic fetal monitor, may trigger an inexorable process that finishes with instrumental delivery or Caesarean section.

Only, of course, it isn't finished. For the woman is left with the impact of the birth experience that changes her self-perception and relationships. This may last a lifetime – women in their seventies have rung me because they needed to talk about a birth that occurred more than 50 years earlier.

In a study of women's long-term memories of their first births Penny Simkin revealed that:

> Women's memories of the events of their births are generally accurate years later despite some lapses or errors in memory of specific details. The significance they attach to negative events seems to intensify and increase over time whereas the positive aspects remain consistently positive in most cases.[5]

It is often claimed that women vie with each other over the awful births they had and that they contaminate pregnant women with fear. In fact, one who has had a traumatic experience is often unwilling to discuss it in front of other women, especially those who are pregnant at the time. She feels isolated, a sort of pariah, who might not only frighten them but, as if from a contagious disease, visit a similar fate on them.

The opposite may happen when members of an antenatal class meet after they have had their babies. Depending on the proportion who have had active management of birth, instrumental deliveries and Caesarean sections, some may compete over the lovely, natural births they had. A woman said:

> No, I haven't talked to any other women about it. You don't want to spoil it for them, do you? The other women in my class all had a very good time. I'm the only one who didn't. It's a bit of a bomb-shell in a conversation to say, 'It was hell, actually . . . the most terrible day of my life.' So I don't say anything – just smile.

Only if their births were complicated are women likely to compete over the degree of trauma they suffered. Either way, other women in the group are silenced.

BIRTH EXPERIENCES

Women who have had both a distressing and a positive birth experience are the ones who speak with greatest clarity to describe the difference between a traumatic and a happy birth. They often contrast a previous birth – an attempt at instrumental delivery (perhaps a botched ventouse, vacuum extractor, delivery and then a forceps delivery, or a failed forceps and then a Caesarean section) – with a recent one – a home birth with one-to-one midwife care.

But sometimes it is the other way around – a peaceful, satisfying first birth followed by one in which they had numerous interventions and felt completely out of control.

They are clear about what caused the contrast. It was not the inherent obstetric characteristics of the labour and delivery but the setting in which they gave birth and the way they were treated: rules, restrictions, rigid protocols, personal neglect, bossiness, unkindness, shift changes and the appearance of nameless strangers – all amounting to fragmented care and disempowerment, and often appalling errors of management or lack of surgical skills.

Occasionally, it is only on looking back that a woman comes to realise that an obstetrician sliced into her rectum, punctured her bladder, cut a blood vessel or nicked the baby's head, or that the anaesthetist misplaced the epidural and penetrated the dura (the fine membrane that surrounds the spinal cord). Nobody told her at the time.

A woman who has experienced a recent satisfying birth sometimes calls Birth Crisis Network to say that she needs to come to terms with an earlier birth which is still going round and round in her mind. She is 'stuck' with it.

In an edition of the serial *The Archers* on BBC radio,[6] an ante-natal class is taking place that is given over to discussion about what the women want. One is determined to have all the pain-killing drugs she can have as soon as she can get them. Another wants a birth without interference and implies that the first is being selfish because she is not considering that the drugs will get through to her baby. 'Who are you calling selfish?' she snaps back. The scene fades and the discussion is picked up again as the prospective parents drive home. The man says, 'It's good to be able to let off steam in a safe and structured environment.' 'Yeeeeeees . . .' the woman replies doubtfully, '. . . until the security services arrived.'

Most antenatal and postnatal discussion groups don't reach that level of altercation. But the programme aptly pinpointed the strong feelings that can be aroused.

WHAT DOES IT MEAN TO BE IN CONTROL OF BIRTH?

The debate about 'control' is challenging because there is little agreement about what the word means. How can you be in control of an elemental force any more than you can control the tides of the sea and the blowing of the wind? A woman who plans to have control over the power of her uterus faces disappointment.

But suppose control means control of pain? There are ways – highly efficient ways with epidural anaesthesia – of controlling pain. Some women believe that if caregivers cannot ensure prompt anaesthesia, they are denying a woman's basic right to freedom of pain in childbirth.

Birth, however, involves much more than pain, and many women discover that the concept of control needs to extend to being able to opt between alternatives, rather than being faced with obstetric ultimatums, and to having control of the environment in which birth takes place.

They often come up against the active management of labour, a system aimed at achieving vigorous obstetric control of labour and birth. It was first introduced in Dublin in the 1960s, and has swept over the world. The bible of active management is a book by O'Driscoll *et al.*[7] Every woman's cervix had to dilate by 1 centimetre per hour (or more) and match a model graph stretching in a steep incline from the lower left-hand corner to the upper right-hand corner of a partogram. If it did not, labour was artificially accelerated. They restricted this management to primigravidae (women giving birth for the first time), were reluctant to induce labour unless urgently necessary, and provided one-to-one care from a student midwife. Today in hospitals internationally, a similar approach is used, together with induction of labour, fragmented and sometimes chaotic care – and it is used on multigravidae (women giving birth to second or subsequent babies) and, sometimes, even on women who have had a previous Caesarean. The rules are:

- *One hour after admission*: artificial rupture of the membranes is performed if the cervix has not dilated by at least 1 centimetre. If the membranes have already ruptured, labour is artificially accelerated.
- *Two hours after admission*: if dilatation is below the line on the graph, labour is artificially accelerated.
- *Three hours after admission*: the time of full dilatation is predicted and the woman is told when she will deliver.

In the National Maternity Hospital Dublin, nurses 'are indemnified against the possibility of cephalopelvic disproportion, rupture of the uterus, and injury to the child . . . Criticism is reserved for those who failed to act decisively to restrict the duration of labour'.[8] They are instructed to:

> *Keep every woman in labour on a tight emotional rein, from the time of admission until her baby is born . . . Women in labour must be encouraged to keep their eyes open at all times because closed eyes usually mask the first step on the road to total disintegration.*[9]

When this is combined with powerful drugs designed to be used for abortion and haemorrhage, continuous fetal monitoring and being tethered to machines, a woman has all control taken from her.

Childbirth becomes torture.

As active management spread around the globe, and in response to the medical autocracy, a new concept was developed concerning patient autonomy – *informed choice*. Simultaneously with the aggressive management of birth, concerns were expressed, first in the US and then in the UK, that child-bearing women should be able to choose how they were cared for, share in all decision-making and have access to the research evidence with which they could evaluate interventions. Women's right to choices became part of the language of childbirth – that was talked about in successive conferences and on innumerable committees much more than it was ever put into practice. Women are misled and feel cheated when, often at the very end of pregnancy or in labour, they discover from health professionals that it is hard to get unbiased information and that there is no real choice.

MAKING AN INFORMED CHOICE

You can explore alternatives in the *Informed Choice* leaflets published by the Midwife's Information and Resource Service (MIDIRS).[10] They provide a good basis for discussion with care-givers as you negotiate what you want. I suggest that you ask for those designed for professionals – not the ones intended for mothers – as they provide evidence and are fully referenced.

Discussion may not be easy if you do not have a midwife who can practise autonomously, and have one who must consult other members of her team before she agrees to anything. When Professor Mavis Kirkham and her researchers studied how the *Informed Choice* leaflets were being used, they encountered midwives who did not encourage any choices that they knew midwifery colleagues would not support. So they avoided discussion about positions and moni-toring. They knew their colleagues would want women to labour in bed and to have continuous electronic monitoring.[11]

You may also come up against stereotyping – being boxed into a category and a set of assumptions about you that makes midwives' work quicker and easier. Women often say to me, 'I don't want to be thought bolshie', 'one of those complaining middle-class mothers' or 'confrontational', and they go out of their way to be compliant, because they think that discussing options is likely to irritate the midwives. It is true that some midwives blame women for taking up time, asking 'too many' questions and disrupting the smooth organisation of the clinic. A midwife in Kirkham's study said:

> *There are a lot of women in my caseload I wouldn't dream of giving the leaflets to . . . like I wouldn't give some of them certain information because I don't want them having certain choices . . . like not having a scan or having the baby at home for instance . . . It would be a complete waste of time giving them leaflets to read.*

She went on to say who these women were: 'Anyway they can't read, a lot of them.'[12]

But professional women with university degrees are often blamed for demanding attention and for being 'stubborn' about having a birth at home, for example, and running what their caregivers believe are unnecessary risks. So the problem is not only the stereotyping of women who are thought to be illiterate, with the aim of both protecting and controlling them, but also controlling educated women who might make a nuisance of themselves. Midwives who approach their patients in this way tend to see these evidence-based leaflets as radical tracts.

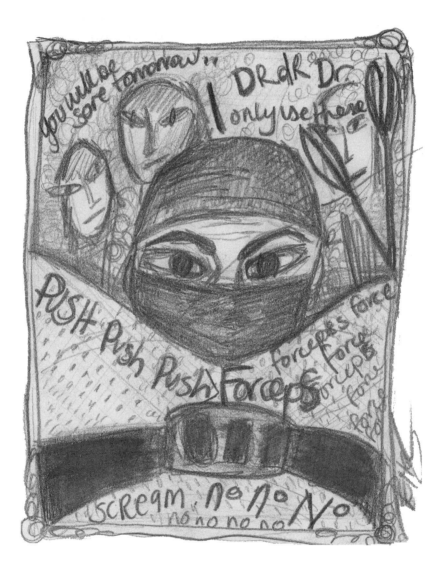

INSTITUTIONAL POWER IN
A HIGH-TECH BIRTH CULTURE

3

HOW AN ANTHROPOLOGIST SEES BIRTH

MANY THINGS DONE TO WOMEN that make childbirth traumatic are not based on research evidence. They are not scientific at all. They are practices through which powerful institutions regulate everything that goes on in them and keep individuals – in the case of hospitals, staff and patients – in line and subservient.

When a woman is admitted to hospital she encounters a social system that regulates her behaviour and that of everyone else in it. There is a bureaucracy designed to ensure conformity and obedience and a hierarchical management structure that punishes deviance and rewards uncritical adherence to the rules and protocols it dictates. This is in dramatic contrast to how birth was in the past.

Historically, giving birth has always been perceived as a major life transition for the woman that reinforces social bonds between families in the community. Traditionally, women came together to define the meaning of each birth for the mother, the baby and the culture as a whole. Medicine, the art of healing, was an element in every woman's household lore, too. All over the world, women have been cared for in childbirth by female friends and a midwife, and the birthplace has been exclusively women's territory.

In medieval Europe a woman summoned her 'god-sibs' – literally sisters-in-god – when she started labour, and the men left the house. Strong drink was consumed by all, including the mother, and though it was acknowledged that birth was a risky process 'there was often more merriment than at a feast'.[13]

The term 'god-sib' changed to 'gossip' as time went on. It offers a clue to how men saw the invasion of the home by the god-sibs and the replacement of male authority. Sienese and Florentine paintings depicting the birth of the Virgin Mary and the birth of St John show scenes of as many as six women helping the mother. They bring her food and drink, and bathe and swaddle the newborn baby. Records from the sixteenth and seventeenth centuries describe how women came with healing herbs and teas to stimulate the uterus and to ease pain, special unguents and balms that were used for massage, alcoholic drink, and sustaining food for after the birth. One woman might also bring the 'Girdle of Mary', a sash, often bright scarlet, that was draped around the mother's pelvis or over her thigh to help the birth through the spiritual power of the Virgin Mary. The local convent might keep a Girdle of Mary to lend out for births in the area, and sometimes it was handed down between women in the family.

In North America, where women were often isolated in farms and rural outposts, they went to great lengths to get female friends and relatives to be with them in childbirth. Women sometimes travelled vast distances to attend and stayed days, or even weeks. When a doctor was present, women friends or family members orchestrated everything that went on within the birth room, and the doctor dared not do anything that met with their disapproval. Young doctors, with little practical experience of birth when they started out in obstetrics, had to attend women in their own homes who were being cared for by other women with a great deal of birth experience and strong opinions about what ought to be done. One doctor said that it was impossible to ensure sterile conditions and 'strip his patient and go at her with soap and scrub brush, lather and razor' because 'there are five or six neighbor women and perhaps, the mother of the patient – all mothers of large families of children.'[14]

The practice of woman-centred and woman-attended births in the home continued, in modified form, well into the twentieth century in rural areas. It was often dangerous to give birth with only a male doctor in attendance, either in hospital – where destitute women went to provide clinical material for doctors learning obstetrics – or outside hospital in a nursing home or at home. In Leeds between 1920 and 1929 three per thousand women died in childbirth in the poorest parts of the city – they were attended by midwives. But in middle-class areas, where doctors attended, six per thousand died. *The Lancet* stated:

> The midwife-employing middle class expect to deliver themselves ... The woman who engages a doctor ... often does so in the expectation that if they do not move quickly the artificial aid that is at hand will be immediately available.[15]

Statistics of maternal deaths in Glasgow and Aberdeen – and, subsequently, national statistics, too – show similar results. Doctors were quick to use the drug pituitrin to speed up a slow labour, and sometimes the result was uterine rupture. They routinely offered chloroform, running the risk of anaesthetic death. They also resorted to forceps delivery, but they often failed to achieve it so they transferred the patient to hospital. In 1929 Henry Jellet, analysing the causes of the high maternal mortality rate, said that doctors had turned 'a physiological process in a healthy woman into a death trap'.[16]

Birth became safer during the Second World War. One reason for this was that the men were away in the armed services, so responsibility for childbirth was reclaimed by midwives, and birth became again, for a brief interval, woman-centred. When men took over again after the war, obstetricians were often eager to try out new technology to show what they could do. As students, they still learned basic skills from midwives, but when they progressed in their careers they concentrated on abnormal and interesting cases, and often never saw another normal labour and birth. It is the same today.

BIRTH PLANS

When a woman presents at the antenatal clinic with a birth plan, it is often shelved and ignored. If she asks a caregiver to look at it when she is in labour midwives may shake their heads and predict that this woman, keen to have a natural birth, is bound to end up with an instrumental delivery or Caesarean. The implication is that because she wants to give birth without drugs she is setting herself up for getting a whole armament of interventions – even that they are going to see to it that she gets them, as if she must be punished for being so foolish for having such high hopes of her birth experience. Women sometimes report that midwives not only fail to discuss their birth plan but laugh about it.

This is sheer bullying. It is similar to ways in which new boys at select boarding schools or recruits in the army are treated. The power of the institution is asserted over the most recent newcomers through its junior members. With threats, humiliation and intimidation they are forced to 'toe the line'.

In a midwives' study of birth plans in one hospital the authors of the study complain that 'birth plans may put pressure on midwives to comply with patients'.[17] They reveal that birth plans irritated the midwives and 'provoked some degree of annoyance' because they were 'unreasonable'. As a result women who made birth plans had more forceps and ventouse deliveries, Caesareans and interventions of every kind.

An Australian study,[18] in contrast, showed that birth plans empowered women – by increasing their knowledge and understanding of birth practices and helping them to make informed choices – and showed the 'commitment of caregivers to recognising and supporting diversity'. In two hospitals 90 per cent of women used birth plans. But even there one third said that they were not encouraged to ask questions. The authors attribute this to the power imbalance between clients and professionals, lack of time, language and cultural barriers and 'embarrassment about appearing ignorant and misinformed'. Yet in the long run, being given enough time to discuss your wishes fully, being able to communicate easily, and feeling that you are treated as a responsible human being all come down to not being overwhelmed by the power imbalance inherent in medicalised childbirth.

Though birth is safer than it ever has been before, for many women today it has become an experience that is disempowering, and the memory haunts them afterwards. The passage to motherhood takes place within a hospital-based technocratic culture and often proves to be a frightening ordeal. Women are physically tethered and psychologically brainwashed, and medical and technological ritual power is asserted and maintained. This happens even when pain is well controlled with an epidural, when there are pictures on the walls, flowery curtains at the windows, a rocking chair, and a patchwork spread on the bed, even when women are persuaded that they have been offered a range of consumer choices and are free to come to their own decisions.

The modern hospital, no less than any traditional society, imposes a culture of childbirth. One aspect of this is being cared for by teams of professional staff rather than by named individuals whom mothers get to know well.

FRAGMENTED CARE

When care is fragmented, a woman's experience of birth is confused, disjointed and shapeless. Fragmented care makes it impossible for a woman to have a personal relationship with her midwife. Giving birth is an intense and intimate experience. Yet the medicalised management of birth turns the labour room into a public arena in which a woman's genitals are exposed to view and anonymous staff members come and go, students observe, strangers examine and monitor progress, and records are handed over as shifts change and new teams come on. A complete stranger may stride into the room, loom over a woman, announce that he is going to 'check' her and then push a gloved hand into her vagina. This system of management is bewildering, humiliating and frightening for the mother. But fragmented care is also dangerous. It creates the conditions for maternal distress, uterine malfunction and prolonged labour. No one takes personal responsibility. Messages are garbled. Snippets of information take the place of understanding. It can be disastrous. One midwife encourages a woman to move around. Then another takes over and insists that she gets back on the bed because that is the only way the fetal heart rate can be monitored properly. With a woman immobilised and lying in a position that make contractions more painful and less effective and that reduces the oxygen flowing to the baby, the fetal heart rate drops. There is general anxiety, an obstetrician is called in, and preparations are made for an instrumental delivery, or the patient is rushed to theatre for a Caesarean section. Or the woman is told that she is 5 centimetres dilated, and then someone else, perhaps with larger fingers, does an internal examination and announces that she is 4 centimetres and that labour must be speeded up because it is taking too long.

THE LANGUAGE OF OBSTETRICS

Today in most countries, with the exception of Russia where most obstetricians are women and have low status in the medical system, birth is men's business. The language of gynaecology and obstet-rics expresses male thought patterns and bristles with images of violence and conquest. This is so for medicine as a whole, too. Medical metaphors derive from military concepts – the body's 'defences', for example – and birth is conducted by 'house officers' who may decide to 'treat aggressively'. Gynaecologists' names are attached to parts of women's bodies and processes of reproduction as if these men had invented them; Fallopian tubes, Bartholin's glands and the Kegel muscle for her pelvic floor.

Birth is defined as an act that is somehow separate from the woman herself – a test, like an exam, at which she either succeeds or fails. If the baby does not engage in a favourable position, it may be because she has an 'inadequate' pelvis. When the cervix is slow to dilate, it is diagnosed as 'incompetent', and 'failure to progress' is recorded in the notes. If she is permitted to attempt a vaginal birth after a previous Caesarean, labour becomes a 'trial of scar'. Even obstetricians who listen to women may talk about 'obstetric performance'. A paper published in the *British Journal of Obstetrics and Gynaecology* that showed that a Caesarean or vaginal instrumental delivery left many women frightened about any future birth and might mean that they avoided getting pregnant again was titled 'Subsequent obstetric performance, related to primary mode of delivery'.[19] If we look at birth as a trial of the uterus or a repro-ductive performance, no wonder many women believe they have failed. We get to see ourselves like rats in an experimental maze.

All 'total' institutions, such as the army, the prison system and large hospitals, have ceremonies and protocols aimed at ensuring safety and develop strategies to keep everyone under control. The medical system manages women in childbirth through enacting rites of passage into motherhood that reinforce the authority of the insti-tution in which birth takes place and that of the doctors and midwives who represent it. A woman is separated from 'normal' people going about their everyday lives. She has routine investigations that entail exposing intimate parts of her body to complete strangers, and is expected to accept anything done to her that is 'for the baby's sake'. The act of birth-giving is defined as a mechanical and technolog-ical process. Uterine contractions and the baby's heart rate are monitored electronically, and a woman's body is treated as if it were a piece of faulty electronic equipment. Instead of receiving one-to-one care from a midwife, the birth-giving is managed and regulated by an obstetric team, the members of which are troubleshooters, data analysts and repair experts.

BECOMING A PATIENT

The system of control starts in pregnancy. A woman becomes a patient. She is subordinated to a complex medical management system. To be a 'good patient' she should be placid, polite, appreciative and quick to respond to instructions and remember what she is told. The word 'patient' derives from 'passivity'. A patient is somebody to whom something is *done*. Interns in an American hospital were asked to define a 'good patient'. One doctor answered, 'She does what I say, hears what I say, believes what I say.'[20] A good patient is dependent and trusting. She is grateful for whatever is done to her. Obstetricians and other professional caregivers still tend to have preconceived ideas about how female patients should behave, often without realising it. A woman who fails to conform is seen as 'a difficult patient'.

Many obstetricians are charming and kind. Some fully support a woman who wants to give birth without drugs and other interventions. But even they are part of a technocratic hospital system that processes women through childbirth. It is hard for them to break away from and to challenge the practices of their colleagues, and also to defend their decision not to intervene when litigation takes place because something has gone wrong and a baby has not survived. Obstetricians often give litigation as the reason why they insist on induction of labour or continuous electronic fetal monitoring, or why they perform a forceps delivery or vacuum extraction or do a Caesarean section. It is 'just in case' obstetrics. In England 47 per cent of births are listed in Department of Health statistics as 'normal' deliveries; 11 per cent are instrumental and 22 per cent are Caesareans.[21] There is often no research evidence for common practices such as routine fetal monitoring, artificial stimulation of the uterus or episiotomy.

When labour starts, or even before it starts, the admission procedure marks the point at which the institution takes control of the woman's body and mind. This is a ceremony in which the woman is registered in the system: the way she should be managed is recorded, her blood pressure is taken, the state of her cervix and degree of dilatation are measured, and the presentation of the baby and the fetal heart rate are recorded. These examinations provide useful information. But they do more than this: they serve as an initiation rite.

Following this, labour is likely to be actively managed. The membranes are artificially ruptured. She is harpooned to a continuous electronic fetal monitor and an intravenous drip that feeds artificial hormone stimulants straight into her blood stream.

She may be allowed nothing to eat, and even fluids may be restricted in case she has a Caesarean section and aspirates stomach contents under general anaesthetic (Mendelson's syndrome). But gastric emptying is slower in labour, and evidence to support this practice is lacking. A woman who does not keep up her blood sugar levels and remain well hydrated is likely to have raised ketone levels and a longer and more painful labour.[22] When intravenous fluids are used instead of allowing her to eat and drink if she wishes, she is not only tethered to a drip and unable to move easily but may be at risk of fluid overload.

CONFORMITY AND PASSIVITY

During childbirth women are controlled by being kept ignorant. They are warned not to listen to other women's birth stories and told to approach birth without any 'preconceived ideas'.

In many hospitals women are separated from friends and family and allowed only one birth partner, who is expected to be the baby's father. They are required to surrender their own clothing, a symbol of individuality, are depersonalised by having to wear a skimpy cotton gown, and may be covered in the delivery room with sterile drapes. They are expected to follow instructions, avoid drawing attention to themselves and be polite and controlled. They are addressed by their first names in a superficially friendly way, but rarely call the obstetrician by his or her first name. In fact, they may not even know the doctor's name at all. Women may lose their names altogether; they may become anonymous and be referred to as 'room 5', 'the Caesarean', 'the multiple birth' or 'the induction'.

In my anthropological work in countries around the world, almost everywhere I have sat with women in labour I have noticed that staff in modern hospitals are most satisfied when they can write on the record sheet 'patient resting peacefully' – whether she is relaxing, is under the influence of narcotic drugs or is quietly moaning and groaning, but *without disturbing anyone else*. I have seen a midwife persuade a woman to accept an opiate injection, not because the woman wanted it but because the midwife said she could not bear to watch her in pain. The ideal patient is tucked in bed, more or less inert. This is one reason why many obstetricians – and midwives, too – like epidurals.

JOKING BEHAVIOUR

Their training prepares budding doctors, and often midwives, to build protective barriers against patients. For doctors this is often reinforced by medical humour, much of which focuses on death and the female body. Humour helps shield them from the reality of human suffering, and also from women's threatening sexuality.

An aspect of any asymmetrical relationship – one between individuals of unequal power – is that the dominant person can engage in licensed familiarity and joking behaviour. When a woman presents a birth plan it may be dismissed with 'You can swing from the chandeliers as far as I am concerned' or – as my own daughter was told when she said she wanted a home birth – 'Deliver on the Headington roundabout if that's what you want'. A midwife standing over a woman writhing in pain laughed and commented, 'It's a bit different from what you were doing nine months ago, isn't it!'

The Italian sociologist Franca Pizzini analysed joking language used with painful interventions in childbirth.[23] She talked about 'privileged offensiveness'. A woman having a repeat Caesarean section recounted how the surgeon cut out the old scar and threw it towards a waste bin – but it fell on the floor, and someone asked, 'Does anyone want it to go fishing?'

A doctor who had just finished suturing a woman's perineum patted her on the leg and exclaimed, 'There you are! Better than new!' Another said, 'Your husband will be really pleased. He will think you are a virgin again.' One who examined an episiotomy made by a subordinate that had extended the tear into the woman's rectum, commented, 'What a dog's dinner!' When a woman was rigid with pain as her cut vulva was swabbed, a nurse smiled and asked, 'Do you act like this when your husband touches you too? Naughty girl! When her husband touches her she is all relaxed, but when we touch her she gets tense!' A woman screamed as a doctor performed a painful manoeuvre and he asked, 'What will your husband think? That I am torturing you? Afterwards he will want to settle accounts with me!'

REALITY IS IN THE CASE NOTES

It is difficult for other doctors to question such behaviour, for the career structure of medicine means that each doctor relies on superiors' and colleagues' approval far more than on what their patients think. The meaning of birth is to be found exclusively in medical records. Women are denied their own definition of birth. If a woman is dissatisfied with what was done to her, or unhappy about how staff behaved, and wants to find out what happened, she must turn to experts and learn *their* construction of events.

Though a brave attempt to do something about the soaring numbers of women who are distressed after having a baby, Birth Afterthoughts schemes in some British hospitals, in which a woman goes through her case notes with a midwife, depend on interpreting the experience in medical terms. The midwife's task is also to soothe and placate, and so prevent litigation. Once events have been explained, it is expected that the patient will be content. Her personal experience may be perceived as uninformed, eccentric, unbalanced, highly emotional – even hysterical. The unhappiness is *her* problem because she suffered childhood sexual abuse, is mentally disturbed, ignorant, self-centred, infantile or had 'unrealistic expectations'.

HARPOONED TO A FETAL MONITOR

The most powerful ritual act practised routinely in labour is wiring up of a woman to a continuous fetal monitor. Research reveals that electronic fetal monitoring (EFM) does not improve outcomes in either low-risk or high-risk mothers, and increases the risk of instrumental delivery and Caesarean section.[24] Yet most women get it. In the US 93 per cent have continuous electronic monitoring.[25]

When a woman is wired to a fetal monitor, information does not come directly from her body and breathing, and from the expression on her face, but from the monitor and other equipment, which may fill the available space – so much so that the woman's partner may not be able to get near her because there is 'no room'. All eyes are on the monitor screen and the uncoiling chart.

There is evidence that electronic fetal monitoring is often employed as a substitute for continuous support.[26] A meta-analysis of nine randomised controlled trials reveals that EFM has not resulted in improved outcomes for babies.[27] And it increases the risk of a Caesarean or instrumental delivery.[28]

This technology gives a powerful message that a woman's body cannot be trusted and is in constant danger of malfunction. Unable to move and change position without interfering with the printout, she is fixed like a specimen studied under bright lights on a lab bench.

CEREMONIAL DRESS

Ceremonial garments are used in religious ceremonies the world over. They depersonalise those wearing them. As labour builds to a climax, if it is an obstetric rather than a midwife birth, a woman may be surrounded by strangers wearing gowns, masks, head covers and overshoes. The function of sterile garments is largely ritual. A mask only prevents the passage of bacteria for about 15 minutes. As long ago as the 1980s *The Lancet* published an editorial that claimed that the wearing of masks 'is no more than an expensive ritual',[29] and a midwife study revealed that infection is reduced on the labour ward when midwives do not wear masks.[30] Sociological research has shown that the higher up in the social hierarchy the individual is, the more often masks were discarded.[31] The senior obstetrician might wander in wearing an ordinary suit and put on sterile clothing only to do an obstetric manoeuvre. The lower the individual in the hierarchy, the more special clothing had to be worn at all times. Yet ordinary cleanliness is often neglected in hospitals, and there are soaring rates of cross-infection because staff do not wash their hands between attending patients and other basic rules of hygiene are ignored.

In many countries, when birth is imminent a woman who is to be delivered by an obstetrician is covered in sheeting. She looks like a sofa draped in dust covers. The only visible object is a plate-sized shiny area of swabbed flesh and a vulva exposed under bright lights. This is called the obstetrician's 'sterile field'. It is a convenient fiction. Because of the juxtaposition of the vulva and the anus, it cannot be sterile. And it is obviously not the obstetrician's. But it is an effective way to depersonalise and desex her genital area.

THE CUT

The final flourish is an episiotomy. This is a ritual mutilation through which many women still pass in order to be mothers. The pain resulting from surgically wounding and then suturing the perineum may persist until the third post-partum month, and often for much longer. Women start out on motherhood *wounded*.

In some countries, after an episiotomy has been performed a manoeuvre is used that entails hooking the baby's chin up by pushing a finger into the women's anus. Fundal pressure with hand grip or elbow pressure may be used to force the head down so this can be done.

Today, midwives in the UK try to avoid performing an episiotomy unless they fear a large tear. Even so, aggressive management of the second stage and the rush to deliver in a birth dominated by the clock puts such pressure on perineal and vulval tissues that an episiotomy may be considered necessary. Thirteen per cent of women who give birth vaginally have an episiotomy.[32] When episiotomies were at their height – and in many British hospitals over 70 per cent of women were being cut – I studied the birth accounts of nearly 2,000 women who had been to National Childbirth Trust classes all over the UK and their experiences of episiotomy and suturing.[33] The alarming thing about episiotomy is that it is a procedure that came into general and almost completely uncritical use without ever being properly evaluated, and without asking women what *they* thought about it. If this can happen with an intervention such as episiotomy, it raises questions about many other obstetric routines.

My research revealed that an episiotomy is more painful than a tear. Thirty-seven per cent of women with episiotomies were in pain at the end of the first week after delivery, compared with 15 per cent of those who tore. They were more likely to find it difficult to get into a comfortable position to hold the baby than those with tears, and to be distracted with pain during breastfeeding. Pain lasted for longer after episiotomy than following a tear and women tended to have more pain when they tried to have intercourse three months after the birth. Twenty-three per cent of those with episiotomies had pain on intercourse, compared with 10 per cent of those who had tears and only 2 per cent of those who had an intact perineum. Most said that they found that nothing helped make intercourse more comfortable except time. Two-thirds had never discussed episiotomy with a doctor or midwife during the pregnancy, and some who had attempted to do so felt fobbed off. Forty-four per cent of episiotomies were performed within half an hour of the start of the second stage, sometimes before the perineum had fully fanned out. Fifty-nine per cent of women said that they were urged to push harder and longer, so that all their concentration was put into pushing instead of opening up. Twenty-two per cent said that they were never told to stop pushing as the head was being born. Some felt that the baby shot out like a cannon ball because they were pushing with all their strength. Seven per cent of women had a double wound, with a tear as well as an episiotomy. These women were in the most pain. They also often had an infection or other problem with healing, and sometimes stitches broke down and they had to be re-sutured. Thirty-seven per cent said they were never given a reason for the episiotomy, either at the time or afterwards. Some said they felt 'violated' or 'mutilated'. Stitching was painful for some women. When they complained, the doctor did not always take any notice, and they might even be told, 'It doesn't hurt. There are no nerve endings there.' In Chapter 4 I look at what is happening in different countries today, discuss the circumstances in which a woman is most likely to have an episiotomy and make suggestions about how to avoid one.

CLEANING UP

Once the baby is born, the umbilical cord is cut immediately, often before it has stopped pulsating, so that the baby does not receive the extra blood from the placenta. Then the placenta is delivered as soon as possible, usually by controlled cord traction. That means pulling on it, but not so hard that the uterus is pulled inside out.

The standard practice in American hospitals attended by large numbers of immigrant and poor women is to pull on the cord while exerting fundal pressure, after which the obstetrician puts an arm up to the elbow into the woman's uterus to 'make sure there is nothing left'. He may use forceps to pull the uterus down to inspect the cervix, too. The woman's body is treated as a machine that must be emptied and examined before allowing it to pass along the assembly line.

To sum up, the delivery room is simultaneously an electronic nerve centre, a theatre in which a medical drama is enacted, and a shrine where the obstetrician is high priest. The management of the second stage represents in microcosm authoritarian control over women in childbirth.

Obstetric skills are valuable in high-risk births, when used with discretion. They can be life saving. But the technocratic management of childbirth – combining technology, critical observation (often by complete strangers), intrusive monitoring and constant interruptions – disturbs the flow of natural hormones that reduce pain and stimulate pleasure and excitement, blocks the spontaneous physiological process, traumatises women and often leaves them not only physically but emotionally damaged. Every intervention – even apparently minor ones, such as rupturing bulging membranes, talking during a contraction, getting a woman up on a bed and encouraging her to push when she has no urge to do so – introduces the need for further interventions – artificial uterine stimulation, painkilling drugs, instrumental delivery or Caesarean section – which increase the possibility of haemorrhage, pelvic infection, a newborn who is admitted to the intensive care nursery, post-natal physical exhaustion, difficulties in breastfeeding – and post-traumatic stress disorder.

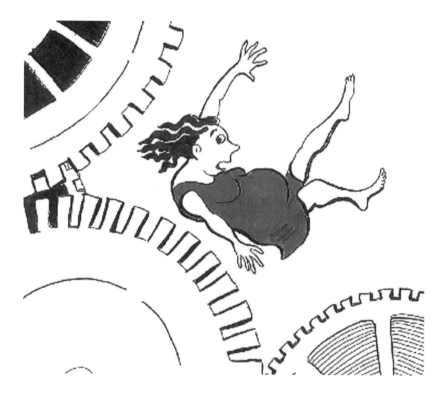

MANAGING THE REPRODUCTIVE MACHINE

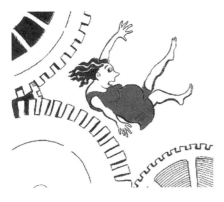

OBSTETRICIANS AND MIDWIVES do not see their actions as ritualised in the way I have described in the previous chapter. They produce explanations for everything they do, based on their perception of a woman's body as being like a machine that must be made to operate efficiently.

The first assumption made in medicalised birth is that our bodies are inherently flawed. They are likely to break down, so those managing them must be alert to forestall malfunction by obstetric interventions to make childbirth conform to a norm. If it is not managed aggressively, there is potential for disaster.

The next assumption – and it leads on from the first – is that our bodies are unaffected by what is going on in our minds (whether we feel free and confident or trapped and anxious, for example) and the interaction between us and other people.

The major decisions about management are to do with 'risk factors'. Every woman is graded 'high' or 'low' risk. It is similar to how eggs are graded on supermarket shelves, but probably less accurate.

There is another important underlying presumption in management: care in childbirth consists in *action*. Negligence consists in failing to intervene, never in intervening unnecessarily.

CLOCK-WATCHED BIRTH

From start to finish birth is regulated by the clock. If labour does not start on the due date, this clock begins ticking. The woman is often allowed several extra days, but if she is not in active labour by a specified date, labour is induced. 'No accurate method, clinical or otherwise, currently exists to determine the onset of labour precisely.'[34] But from the point when a woman is admitted to hospital, or when there happened to be the first vaginal examination, if her cervix fails to dilate by 1 centimetre each hour, the uterus is artificially stimulated. Birth is managed according to a production timetable. Uterine activity has to comply with a superimposed schedule, and if there is deviation from it, synthetic oxytocin is introduced into the mother's bloodstream through an intravenous drip. In many hospitals one is set up 'just in case' so that other drugs can also be fed into her circulation, prostaglandin gel is pushed up into her cervix, or prostaglandins are given orally. If she has not delivered within a predetermined time after the cervix is assessed as fully dilated, whether or not she has any spontaneous urge to push, a ventouse or forceps delivery is performed – or there are attempts at both – or the decision is made to do a Caesarean section.

The obstetrician who introduced the 'Labour Curve' to measure normal progress was Emmanuel Friedman. He did this in 1954, and it has remained the norm by which to measure labour ever since, except that the time allowed for expulsion has been reduced by many obstetricians from the two hours that he stated was the normal limit to one and a half hours, one hour, three-quarters of an hour, or even less.

The partogram provides a sharp visual image of this. It is a line from the bottom left corner of graph paper to the top right.

Commenting on 'straight line thinking, exemplified by this demarcation and quantification', Kirsten Baker, a midwifery lecturer at the University of the West of England, writes, 'Given the phallic symbolism of the upwards sloping line depicting progress in labour, small wonder that there is anxiety when the line deviates from straight.'[35]

A midwifery study of 419 nurse-assisted or midwife-assisted labours revealed that the second stage could last as long as eight hours from dilatation of the cervix in some cases and still be normal, with no adverse affects for the mother and baby.[36] Yet in most births tight protocols are in force, and a woman must push out her baby within the imposed time limits if delivery is not to be by ventouse, forceps or Caesarean section. We ought to ask searching questions about these imposed time limits, and research into the *range of the normal* needs to be conducted urgently.

A RACE TO THE FINISHING POST

A characteristic of traumatic birth experiences, with very few exceptions, is that labour is actively managed and clock-watched, and many interventions take place as a result. These are often done without discussion with the woman, and without giving her accurate information. She has no choice.

The cervix must dilate 1 centimetre each hour or the uterus is failing in its task. The patient must push the baby out in the prescribed time. Once pelvic examination indicates that her cervix is fully dilated, everything must happen at top speed. Birth is treated as a race to the finishing post. Attention is directed to emptying the uterus as speedily as possible. In some Eastern European countries it is the rule that all deliveries must be done by an obstetrician, so nurses prepare the patient and position her, swab her perineum with antiseptic, lay out instruments and tether her legs and fix them to lithotomy stirrups to make the obstetrician's task easier. But even in a midwife-conducted birth all eyes are usually fixed on the bulging perineum and the offending orifice. It is like anxiously watching for your luggage to appear on the carousel at the airport. The woman is coaxed, commanded and often bullied to push strenuously and hold her breath as long as she can. Her cheerleaders urge her to push harder and longer. 'Take a deep breath and hold it and push!' 'Try harder! You can do better than that!' 'Push as if you're constipated!' – even 'Get angry with the baby!'

This kind of pushing leads to fluctuations in the woman's blood pressure and is likely to reduce the oxygen flowing to the baby. It registers on the monitor as 'type 2' dips in the fetal heart rate – ones that continue after a contraction is over. The result is renewed efforts to get the mother to push more energetically, an episiotomy, and if that does not work, an instrumental delivery or emergency Caesarean.

INDUCTION

In the 1970s every second woman giving birth in Britain had her labour induced. Then research was published that showed that these rates of induction introduced unnecessary risks.[37] Rates dropped but are now climbing again. Only two-thirds of women who are induced deliver spontaneously. Fifteen per cent have instrumental deliveries and 19 per cent have emergency Caesarean sections.[38] Chalmers showed that there was an association between the administration of oxytocin for induction or acceleration of labour and jaundice in the baby. A baby whose mother has oxytocin is at 1.6 times greater risk of developing jaundice.[39]

Artificially revving up the uterus tends to make labour more painful, too. Midwives realise this, and some advise a woman to have an epidural *before* these drugs are introduced. Doctors do not always acknowledge that an induced or speeded-up labour may be more painful. Even if it proves to be excessively painful, some consider that it is because the woman had unrealistic expectations of a natural birth, that the pain is nothing to do with the way the labour was managed, and that it was the woman's attitude that produced it. I have heard one German obstetrician claim that such pain was largely 'an organic correlate of unconscious feelings of guilt'.[40]

Back in the late 1970s I studied the experiences of some women who had been to National Childbirth Trust classes. Of these women, 641 were induced and 224 started labour spontaneously. All were highly motivated to have as few drugs as possible. Yet I discovered that only 8 per cent of those who had an induced labour were able to handle it without painkilling drugs, whereas 50 per cent coped without drugs in spontaneous labour.[41]

I wrote articles about this in the national press and women's magazines, and spoke on radio. Women began to share with each other their often highly negative experiences of induced labour. Some obstetricians claimed that their strong, sometimes angry, reactions to induction had been artificially engineered by the media, and even by the research into induction that had begun. Induction was 'enhanced' labour. These women's experiences could not be 'real'. One senior obstetrician wrote:

> *I do not believe that we are seeing other than the response of a relative vocal minority of the patient population. If the vast majority were not encouraged by the media, and by question-naires, to express disappointment and frustration and discontent, they could be effectively dealt with.*[42]

At the onset of the twenty-first century the induction rate in the UK was 20 per cent and in some hospitals, the Princess Royal in Glasgow, for example, it was as high as 40 per cent.

Induction of labour is a major factor for most women who seek help in distress about their birth experiences. Of 500 women who rang me to talk about their traumatic births, nine out of ten had had their labours induced. Many had had failed inductions that culminated in instrumental delivery, failed instrumental delivery and/or Caesarean section.

Unless a woman has had early pregnancy ultrasound it is difficult to work out the expected date of delivery (EDD) with accuracy. The date of the last menstrual period (LMP) is likely to overestimate the length of pregnancy.[43] Her periods may not have been absolutely regular. She may have been on the Pill or just come off it. Or she may not be really sure of the date. Doctors and midwives guess the due date with 'Naegele's rule', reckoning that every pregnancy lasts 280 days from the first day of the last period, that periods come in a 28-day cycle, and that on day 14 ovulation occurred. This usually results in a date earlier than it really is. Add *at least three days*.[44]

There is a slightly increased risk to a baby born after the forty-second week of pregnancy, but if it has been growing well in the uterus, this is minimal. Though the discussion that takes place between a woman and her obstetrician is all about relative risk. It should be noted that, for the group of women who have not yet reached 42 weeks, 500 inductions are done to avoid one perinatal death.[45]

In the 1980s the World Health Organization (WHO) recommended an induction rate of 10 per cent or less.[46] In the US rates were above 19 per cent in 1996, compared with 9 per cent in 1986. That was excluding artificial rupture of the membranes, another way of trying to initiate labour. Not only were there more inductions but they took place earlier, and there were more for post-maturity and large-for-dates fetuses. Caesarean sections after induction went up from 0.7 per cent in 1980 to 4.1 per cent in 1995. Prostaglandins were introduced to stimulate labour, and there were often repeated attempts at induction, and other interventions.[47] The US Listening to Mothers survey of 2002 revealed that 44 per cent of women experienced attempts at induction, but these were successful only one third of the time.[48]

There is a regularly repeated pattern of events that instil fear:

- Concern that a woman has gone past her due date causes her anxiety, and a conviction that her body is not working as it should.
- Induction signifies crisis. It implies that the baby is at heightened risk, and means that labour is taken out of her hands. From now on she has no control over what happens.

Admission to hospital for induction may entail being transferred from a group of midwives she has come to know to a team of caregivers who follow the instructions of an obstetrician. Midwives may be unhappy about an obstetrician's decision to induce. One midwife called me about a woman who had had her labour induced at 39 weeks on Christmas Eve, 'because they didn't want her to have her baby on Christmas Day'.

There are women who welcome induction. Some are so exhausted at the end of pregnancy that they see it as an escape from an intolerable burden. Some ask for labour to be induced because they have been told that an overdue baby is at risk. A woman who was 10 days past her due date was warned by the doctor that she must agree to induction or 'the baby will die'. Prostaglandins were introduced, and when labour failed to start they were given in increasingly large doses. The baby was delivered by forceps after 59 hours of 'chemically induced contractions that I couldn't handle'. She had 'a bit of a breakdown' five months after the birth and called me when her baby was nine months old and she was still having nightmares. She said, 'When that doctor told me I was killing my baby I should have told her to go stuff herself.'

Women who are themselves in nursing or medicine may be even more anxious about this. One woman, a nurse, pressed for induction, which was attempted on day 11 after the expected due day, but failed. Prostaglandins were introduced repeatedly until she finally went into labour on day 16. By this time she was exhausted. Her uterus was overstimulated. The baby was in poor condition and would not feed, 'went blue' and 'nearly starved to death'.

There are women who want the certainty of knowing when the birth will take place, because their partners are available only at that time, or because child care can be booked in advance. Some are anxious to get labour started because the birth must fit in with the timetable of someone who has arranged to come to care for them once the baby is born, or to avoid their mothers being at the birth, but wanting them to come the following week.

Or women may press to be induced for much more serious reasons. Women in the Occupied Palestinian Territories who must line up to pass through Israeli checkpoints before they can get to an Israeli hospital may choose induction to avoid the anxiety of not knowing whether they can make it to the hospital. Some give birth in the open without assistance, watched by soldiers. For them, induction or elective Caesarean section is preferable. Induction and Caesarean rates have shot up for women living in the Gaza Strip.[49]

A woman may ask to be induced because she has had a previous pregnancy in which her baby was diagnosed at risk or she has lost a baby. One woman requested induction at 36 weeks because her first baby had been stillborn and her second baby was diagnosed as growth retarded at 34 weeks. The second labour had been induced and the baby 'was born within 3 hours and he was absolutely fine and I was out the next day'. When she asked to be induced with her third baby 'they told me he was fine and there was no real reason to induce'. She managed to persuade the obstetrician, had a traumatic labour, and rang me because she was having nightmares, waking up trying to pull off an oxygen mask, and was being treated for post-natal depression. Her distress about this birth and her insistence on induction was related to her anxiety during pregnancy about her second baby and the stillbirth of her first.

A disabled woman told me that she had intermittent bleeding. It started at 13 weeks and her membranes ruptured prematurely at 25 weeks when she was out shopping for baby clothes. She was rushed to hospital, where she was given steroids to help the baby's lungs develop. Three weeks later she started bleeding again and labour was induced. She welcomed the decision:

The midwife was just talking openly about the fact that I'd only got a 50/50 chance of surviving . . . All I wanted was just this thing out of my body and I wished I had never been pregnant. I was so scared!

MISOPROSTOL

The effect of drugs administered to induce labour is often not known, and some have not been licensed for this purpose. One such drug, manufactured by Searle in the US, is Misoprostol (Cytotec in the US). It is a form of prostaglandin. Once a drug has been approved for any specific use by the US Federal Drugs Administration, it is legal to prescribe it for other medical conditions. Misoprostol is used for termination of pregnancy; it evacuates the uterus thoroughly and controls post-partum haemorrhage. It started to be used for induction of labour on the basis of evidence that it emptied the uterus of its contents and very efficiently clamped down on it afterwards. Data on Misoprostol induction are not collected, so we cannot know how many labours are kick-started in this way. All synthetic prostaglandins subject the uterus to the risk of hyperstimulation. For both the mother and the baby the risk appears to be greatest when Misoprostol is introduced into the cervix.[50]

Midwives are aware of the powerful and sometimes devastating effects of Misoprostol. In one hospital they refer to it as 'the bomb'. It can cause uterine hyperstimulation, fetal distress and even uterine rupture:[51] This is what often happens when a woman has Misoprostol:

- Violent contractions may suddenly start and overwhelm the woman. She is in shock.
- The process of induction is sometimes prolonged. Induction is started, stopped and then started again. The woman becomes exhausted.
- Continuous fetal monitoring usually entails immobilisation.
- The woman suffers intense pain which is exacerbated if she must be in a reclining position.
- Pain becomes distress. She feels she cannot cope any more. She may feel that she is going to die.
- Drugs for pain relief are given because contractions are sharp and close together.
- An epidural is offered. It provides good pain relief. But there are side effects. It tends to make labour longer by about an hour, so uterine activity is further augmented with drugs.
- The baby's heart rate drops temporarily and fetal distress is diagnosed.
- Deep transverse arrest occurs.
- Attempts at ventouse delivery fail. Forceps delivery may be effective, or forceps may fail too.

- Emergency Caesarean is performed. At birth the baby has a low Apgar score (under 7), and both mother and baby have a raised temperature, so there are investigations to reveal whether this is due to infection. Antibiotics may be prescribed.

In the script of induced labour, physiological and psychological elements are intertwined. Labour is kick-started, so there is the impact of an artificially triggered and usually speeded-up process. The woman submits to this for the sake of her baby. Having her body treated like a failed machine is bound to affect her birth experience. Suddenly she is not a healthy woman giving birth but a patient, passive and receiving treatment aimed at salvaging a baby at risk of brain damage and death. The sense of having personal control in childbirth is fundamental if she is to look back on the experience as positive. Lack of control is a major risk factor for a negative experience.[52,53] To be confident in herself and feel in control, a woman needs support – not just reassurance and sympathy, but support to have her own space, make her own decisions, and do what she feels like doing.

For many women induction of labour represents in an acute way complete loss of control over birth giving. Once that happens, all other interventions are further evidence of simply being on the receiving end of care.

Induction of labour abruptly changes the relationship between a woman and her caregivers, too. Before, they may have appeared to be co-operating with her to have the kind of birth she wants. Once the decision is made to induce, even if she consents without feeling under pressure to do so, power is in their hands. Women are often persuaded to consent. The obstetrician says, 'You don't want to lose your baby, do you?' Persuasion, however, may not be necessary – the obstetrician needs only to hint that resistance on the women's part indicates that she is being selfish. So a woman's perception of her body and her ability to give birth is changed, the relationship with those caring for her is changed, and the physiology of birth is changed dramatically. It is the interaction between these three elements that results in trauma and distress.

SUGGESTIONS TO AVOID UNNECESSARY INDUCTION

- Choose one-to-one midwife care if it is available.
- The best – and sometimes the only – way to have a midwife whom you get to know is to find a birth centre or an independent midwife.

- Before registering with a consultant team, find out the policies and protocols.
- Ask the senior registrar or consultant to tell you the induction rate over the last two years. Have pen and paper ready and note the information. If the answer is vague or seems evasive, ask if accurate figures are available. If this is the case, ask if they can be sent to you in a letter, or if you can make another appointment to receive them.
- Before registering, ask the midwife at the hospital different consultants' policies and practices regarding induction. Don't write this down. Simply have a discussion together. You can probably get some clues.
- Get in touch with other women who have given birth at this hospital and ask them if they can tell you about their experience of induction, and find out which consultant teams were involved. You may be able to do this best through contacts in your antenatal class, friends and friends of friends.
- Seek advice from your local National Childbirth Trust (NCT) or Active Birth teacher.
- If you go past your 'due date', you may agree to monitor the baby's well-being by cardiotocograph (CTG), Doppler ultrasound or some other simple, non-invasive technique of assessing the fetus. Stay sensitively aware of how the baby is moving – how, where (feet, knees, head or body roll) and when. An active baby is likely to be a healthy one.
- If you are considering induction, ask if your cervix is ripe. A ripe cervix suggests that an induction is more likely to be successful. On the other hand, Misoprostol is so powerful that it should *not* be used on a ripe cervix. You can probably tell if your cervix is ripe. Squat down and push two fingers in your vagina. If you feel something like the tip of your nose deep inside, the cervix is not ripe. If you feel a soft mass like a squashy plum, it is ripe. Misoprostol is also dangerous when used on an already scarred uterus.
- The Royal College of Obstetricians and Gynaecologists (RCOG) recommends that women should be offered a membrane sweep before performing an induction. Popping the bubble in which the baby is nestled may be enough to start labour.[54] This can be followed with prostaglandin induction if necessary. On the other hand, even without a membrane sweep, prostaglandins are likely to be effective.

Formal policies and protocols do not always correspond with practice. You will learn this as you research the subject. Mr A, who is a charmer and 'very good with patients', may ask, 'When would you like to have your baby?' Miss B is 'no nonsense' and routinely induces at term +7 days, warning women of the risks to the baby if they do not consent. Mr C prefers to induce at term +4 or 5 days, but not if it is the weekend or he is otherwise engaged, and not in August and Christmas because the hospital is short staffed. Mr D tends to get into conflict with women who do not wish to be induced, then becomes dismissive, and lets the woman take the responsibility, but is apt to make no arrangements to monitor the baby's condition by CTG (ultrasound). Mr E has little confidence in how women's bodies work and prefers routine induction at 38 weeks. He has a high Caesarean section rate. But that is partly because the senior registrar hasn't got the hang of the ventouse (vacuum extractor) so women have a failed ventouse, followed by forceps. When forceps fail, too, there is a 'crash' Caesarean. Mr F believes an elective Caesarean is a wise choice because 'it's better to be safe than sorry'. He also cites studies that show high rates of pelvic floor and bladder damage following vaginal birth. The evidence is flawed, since these labours often had massive interventions, and their effects on the birth were not taken into consideration.

If you are not satisfied with the information you get, you can change consultants, change hospital or switch from consultant to total midwife care.

AMNIOTOMY

Most women can expect to have their membranes ruptured artificially if the waters do not break before or at the beginning of labour. Amniotomy is often performed without discussion or consent. It sometimes occurs by mistake with vaginal examination – sometimes, too, 'by mistake on purpose' by a midwife who wants to hurry labour on. If after amniotomy labour does not speed up, the mother is under pressure to accept drugs to stimulate the uterus. Contractions may get stronger and closer together following artificial rupture of the membranes (ARM), and women are often unprepared for the greater intensity. Once the amnion and chorion are ruptured there is increased urgency to deliver within a stated time span, because the removal of the protective sac in which the baby is lying exposes the baby to infection if labour is long and there are repeated vaginal examinations. Women are often aware of this and feel they have to 'perform'. With artificial rupture of the membranes a labour that was previously relaxed and unforced becomes actively managed.

It is worth discussing this with your midwife and making it quite clear if you do not wish to have amniotomy until your cervix is at least half dilated. The usual natural pattern is for membranes to rupture towards the end of the first stage.

Thus something that seems to many caregivers to be a minor intervention that takes place more or less routinely can change the whole character of the labour and trigger other obstetric interventions. Women are rarely informed of this.

Both induction of labour and amniotomy without consent are acts of assault and may compound other assaults. Anne, with a history of sexual abuse, had an unexplained stillbirth. Knowing that her baby would not be born alive, she wanted a home birth, but her independent midwife said she must be admitted to hospital. Labour was induced with Misoprostol without discussion. This resulted in uterine hyperstimulation. She was unable to give informed consent because alternatives were never discussed with her. She asked to be cared for by female staff and went into hospital with her independent midwife, who felt that she could not interfere with hospital protocol or challenge practice in any way, so she simply held her client's hand and tried to calm and reassure her. Anne says, 'I desperately needed protecting and I am devastated that I had to endure an ever changing succession of medical staff repeatedly invading my body.' She describes the amniotomy:

> Having agreed to allow a midwife to examine me instead of a male doctor, she totally betrayed my trust by sweeping my membranes without consent. She caused me considerable pain and I was frightened. It was the first time that Pete was not present to support me. In his absence I put my trust in the independent and the hospital midwife, and found myself being assaulted.

EPISIOTOMY

As with other interventions in childbirth, the practice of episiotomy seems to be less to do with the mother's or the baby's needs than with custom and professional opinion. It is not based on research evidence.

Rates of episiotomy range from 9.7 per cent in Sweden to 100 per cent in Taiwan.[55] The US rate is 32.7 per cent, whereas it is 11 per cent in Australia and 13 per cent in England. Many episiotomies are unnecessary.

Episiotomy is more likely when there is an instrumental delivery and when a woman has an epidural.[56] There are wide variations in episiotomy rates between different caregivers, sometimes even in the same hospital. A study in Dublin revealed that it ranged from 6 per cent to 84 per cent.[57] Women are also more at risk of having an episiotomy if they have a private obstetrician.[58] In the US they are less at risk if they are on Medicaid.[59]

Many women for whom episiotomy and its after-effects are traumatic have a wound that is extended into a laceration resulting in a third-degree tear (called fourth-degree in the US). They have intense perineal pain after the birth, sometimes for months, and the wound does not heal well and becomes infected. They say it feels as if they are sitting on thorns imbedded in tender flesh, jagged glass or spikes. It hurts to move and to pick up, hold and breastfeed the baby. Many need repair surgery. The reason why a woman may prefer elective Caesarean section to vaginal birth is perineal trauma suffered after a previous vaginal birth. One woman described the after-effects of her episiotomy this way:

I waited 3 hours to be stitched up and the doctor who did it was groaning and muttering about being woken up and what a mess it was. 'What a bloody jigsaw' she said. When I complained about the pain she looked up and said sharply, 'What do you expect?' Then she gave up and called a senior doctor who had to take all the stitches out and had to do them again. It was 18 months before I could sit on my bike.

Another told me:

They just stood talking about other things over me while they stitched me up. It was incredibly painful. I couldn't keep still and they got upset with me. Then they wrote in red on my notes, 'Uncooperative during suturing'. I can still feel it like burning. They left me feeling like I had messed the whole thing up . . . I feel a total failure.

Whether or not a woman gets a routine episiotomy, and the degree of skill with which the wound is sutured afterwards, tend to be 'the

45

luck of the draw', depending on where she lives and the hospital and the obstetrician she selects or happens to get. Many women have no choice and little or no information on which to base any choice.

HOW TO AVOID AN EPISIOTOMY

- Explore the possibility of one-to-one midwife care.
- Plan a home or birth-centre birth.
- Choose care from midwives rather than a private obstetrician.
- Discuss with whoever is going to care for you their policy on episiotomy.
- Following this discussion, record your wishes in your birth plan.
- Consider giving birth in a pool if you have the option. There is some evidence that birth in water reduces pressure on the perineum.[60]
- Let whoever is attending you at the birth know that you would like to avoid an episiotomy and prefer a tear to a cut.
- Massage your perineum with a vegetable or nut oil each day during the second half of pregnancy. As you do so, think about the tissues fanning out and opening up. With your fingertips just inside your vagina, press down on the edge nearest your anus, imagining it as the pressure of the baby's head, and respond to the sensation by relaxing all the muscles around it.
- Wait to push until you cannot avoid doing so. Then push only when, as long as and as strongly as you wish.
- Breathe whenever you can.
- Greet each contraction with a long breath out. Then breathe as you want to. Give another long breath out at the end of each contraction, and relax completely.
- Ask whoever is helping you in the second stage of labour to let you push when and how you like, and not give you instructions or persuade you to push harder and longer than your spontaneous urge.
- Find a comfortable position and change it as you want to.
- Keep your spine and pelvis flexible.
- Let the power of your uterus sweep through you. Do not resist it. And do not force it.
- Avoid deliberate prolonged breath-holding and breathe when you wish.

- Focus on relaxing and opening up as you push.
- Welcome the sensation of stretching to your utmost. It means that your baby is being born and will soon be in your arms.
- When you feel the pressure of your baby's head on your perineum release the muscles of your lower face and throat.
- *Breathe* your baby out, rather than pushing it out.
- Stop pushing, drop your jaw, and breathe in and out through your mouth when the midwife tells you, so that the baby's head can be born gently. If you can, *breathe* out the baby's head rather than pushing it out.

HOW A MIDWIFE CAN HELP

- Trust the mother, and support her in trusting what her body tells her to do.
- Create an environment that is quiet and beautiful, in which lights are low, and in which no one intrudes.
- Avoid stimulating the uterus artificially.
- Do not tell the mother when and how to push. Wait for the spontaneous urge.
- Do not tell her to hold her breath.
- Help her into any position which she feels is right, and help her to change position if she wants to.
- Let her know she is doing well. Encourage her with your eyes, smile, and gestures. If you speak, keep your voice low.
- Avoid vaginal examination if you can.
- If the mother is confident and in tune with contractions, and the perineum is fanning out, consider *not* guarding the perineum. Help her focus on opening.
- Remind her that you will tell her to stop pushing and start breathing with open mouth as the baby's head is crowning.
- Unless you need to intervene, let the baby's head be born slowly and gently without counter-pressure.
- If the mother wants to touch the baby's head as it bulges on the perineum and/or to see it in a mirror held at the right angle, this may help her cope with the sensations.

THE PARTNER

- Give quiet encouragement.
- Offer physical support.
- Use a cold compress on her brow between contractions.
- Between contractions offer ice or a cold sponge to suck, or water through a bendy straw.
- Between contractions massage her back, the back of her head, the small of her back, or her feet if she likes it. Be guided by her.

THE DOULA

A doula is a hired companion who gives constant support through birth. She does not replace a partner but supports you both if that is what you would like.

- Before labour starts, rehearse long, low-pitched breaths out, while releasing the perineum.
- Offer the mother ice chips or sponge to suck, and sips of cold water.
- Mop her brow with a cold cloth.
- Support her shoulders and head if she wants it.
- Between contractions massage her head, shoulders, feet, lower back, buttocks or the outside of her thighs slowly and firmly – whatever she says helps.
- Aim for a good relationship with the midwife.
- Be aware of the partner's needs and give support.
- Indicate how the partner can help. He/she may want to do something active: give physical support, mop her brow with an ice-cold cloth, caress her, stroke and massage her, look into her eyes. It depends on what the mother wants. It may be enough that her partner is simply there.
- If the mother starts to scream, suggest making sounds more like a cow mooing.
- As the head crowns, open your mouth, let your own jaw drop and breathe out in sighs. This is the only guidance she may need. It doesn't matter if she cannot see you doing this.

WHY MESS ABOUT? THE 'NO INDICATED RISK' CAESAREAN

In the US more than 26 per cent of women have Caesarean sections. The primary Caesarean rate for exceptionally low-risk women rose 67 per cent between 1991 and 2001.[61] Of women over 24, 19.5 per cent had a 'no indicated risk' primary Caesarean in 2001. They had the operation because they were considered 'old'. The odds of having a 'no indicated risk' primary Caesarean were nearly 50 per cent higher than the odds for comparable mothers in 1996.[62] The reasons for this are partly – maybe predominantly – economic.[63] Elective Caesarean delivery is simpler to plan for and manage than normal childbirth with all its uncertainties. Maternity care is big business. To run a business efficiently and cover high overhead costs you need a continuous operational flow. Hospital income is increased by induction of labour, active management, electronic fetal monitoring (to reduce staffing, since one observer can monitor several mothers and babies at a time at the central nursing station), epidurals, a range of state-of-the-art technology that is used to attract customers, and neonatal intensive care units to which babies who are not ill are admitted. Private hospitals bill patients for all these extra interventions. Caesarean section rates continue to rise and in November 2003 26 per cent of US women were giving birth by Caesarean.

A planned Caesarean can be performed in only 20 to 30 minutes and scheduled conveniently around office hours. Labour, in contrast, takes hours or days and is unpredictable. There is no question that planned Caesareans are more profitable both for the obstetrician and for the hospital.[64]

In profit-making obstetrics, planned Caesareans appeal to doctors, since they can fit in more patients who take less time to manage and are more under control than those who go into labour haphazardly (and often at inconvenient times), and in whom the length of labour cannot be predicted. Patients, or their insurance companies, pay more for this service.

In the UK it is one reason why women who choose a private obstetrician are much more likely to have a Caesarean than those who have care within the National Health Service (NHS) – a pattern repeated around the world wherever a not-for-profit health system exists alongside obstetrics for profit.[65,66] Caesareans make sense for hospitals that are run as businesses. Operations can be scheduled to make the most efficient use of staff, equipment and other resources.[67]

The US style of obstetric care is contagious and quickly spreads to other countries, even developing ones, where a high dependence on technology and multiple obstetric interventions are attractive to doctors and hospital managers.

Side effects of Caesarean section

A Caesarean can be life saving for a baby. It can prevent a baby being born with brain damage and save the mother from a complicated instrumental delivery or – especially in countries such as Africa, where women who really need them cannot get Caesareans – from death as a result of obstructed labour. But most Caesareans are performed for less pressing reasons.

The risks are rarely discussed in the media. Very few women die after a Caesarean. Yet even for planned Caesareans the death rate is twice that for vaginal birth.[68] The Report of the Confidential Enquiries into Maternal Deaths in the UK reveals that the leading factors are hypertension, thrombosis, sepsis, haemorrhage, amniotic fluid embolism and anaesthesia:[69]

- Women are more at risk of inflammation of the lining of the uterus after a Caesarean than a vaginal birth.
- Some need to have a blood transfusion.
- They are more likely to get pneumonia.[70]
- If the next labour is induced with prostaglandins or Misoprostol introduced into the cervix there is a much-increased risk of uterine rupture.[71,72,73]

We don't know much about the long-term effects of Caesarean birth on babies, but when one is performed before labour starts naturally the baby is bound to be born earlier than it would have been and to be of lower weight;[74] Caesarean babies are also more likely to have breathing problems.[75] After an elective Caesarean up to 1 in 18 compared with 1 in 63 babies born vaginally need oxygen and mechanical ventilation.[76]

A woman should not have a Caesarean just because her baby is big. This applies when she has had a previous Caesarean, too.[77,78] She is likely to face fewer health problems with a vaginal birth after a previous Caesarean than if she automatically has more surgery.[79]

ACTION A PREGNANT WOMAN CAN TAKE

- If an elective Caesarean is suggested, ask why.
- Ask for references to evidence-based research – randomised controlled trials – related to this.
- Ask for alternative care options and research evidence concerning these, too.
- Say you need time to think about it. Use this time to research the subject and discuss it with anyone who is going to help you in childbirth. Consult relevant organisations and websites listed in the 'Useful addresses' (pp. 169–73).
- If you are not convinced by the evidence, put your decision in writing to the obstetrician and state clearly what you would prefer.

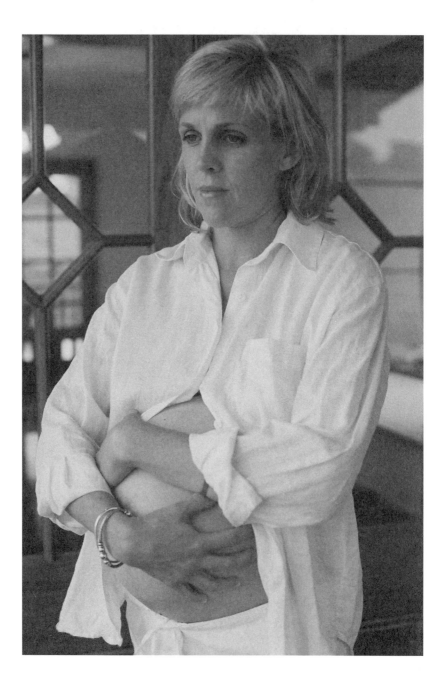

SEXUAL ABUSE AND BIRTH

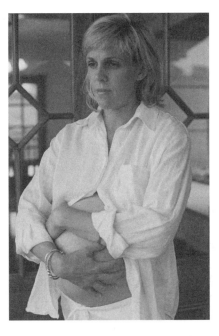

We were catheterising an old, blind woman; she must have been about 90. It took four nurses to carry out the procedure – three of us were needed to hold her down. And all this old woman was saying was: 'Please don't do it daddy, please don't do it daddy.' We all went silent. It was never discussed, nobody dared mention it.[80]

THE NURSE DESCRIBING THIS INCIDENT told my daughter Jenny that she was distressed that there was no support either for the woman or the staff.

For some women, medical procedures in pregnancy and birth bring back overwhelming memories of sexual violence, events they had pushed into the back of their minds and apparently forgotten. Jenny interviewed 39 survivors of childhood sexual abuse and wrote articles to help doctors, nurses and midwives understand how to 'counteract, not re-enact the violation of women's bodies'.[81]

She described how the experience of sexual abuse affected gynaeco-logical examinations, pregnancy and birth. More than half of them had flashbacks. Internal examinations, cervical smears and even dental examinations reminded them of the sexual assaults: 'The action of inserting a speculum into the vagina or fingers into the mouth can remind women of vaginal or oral rape. The experience of being helpless in the hands of another person recalls their power-lessness during abuse.' One abuse survivor told Jenny that her father used to tie her up. When she was in labour, she was 'spread-eagled on a bed, my arms tied to drips, someone fiddling around down there – it brought back the bondage.' It is hardly surprising that she says she 'flipped'.

No one knows how many children are sexually abused. It depends on how abuse is defined and the sensitivity of the research tool. Estimates in the US go as high as 55 per cent. In an article written for childbirth educators, Penny Simkin points out that:

> *The true rate for either sex is impossible to determine, given the secrecy, shame, and guilt many children and survivors carry with them as a result of the abuse, and given the threats to remain silent often imposed on them by their abusers.*

She states: 'It is likely that every childbirth class includes survivors of sexual abuse.'[82] It means that every midwife and every doula will also encounter abuse survivors among their clients.

We all know what it is like to be powerless as children: being dictated to, overruled and dominated. That is not an experience restricted to women who have been sexually abused. Women who have been abused as children are not 'special cases' to be treated differently from other women.

Nor should it be assumed that every woman who has been sexu-ally abused requires therapy. For many women it has increased their understanding of issues of power and powerlessness in the health services. They are not gullible and they know how to negotiate what they want. Nor do they wish to be labelled. They are survivors, not victims.

A survivor may have no recollection of abuse, but an intense memory suddenly overwhelms her as she has a gynaecological exam-ination or is in labour. The memory of abuse is often repressed. Amnesia is one way of surviving.

In her book *My Father's House: A Memoir of Incest and Healing*, Sylvia Fraser said:

We tend to think of memory as only residing in the mind, but the body has specific memories too. My body remembered what my mind forgot, and when the memories came back, they came back as convulsions – the convulsions of a child being orally raped.[83]

A woman may panic when she is put into the same position as that in which she was usually abused – lying flat on her back, perhaps, or on her side, because that is how she lay, pretending to be asleep, while she was abused from behind. If her movement is restricted in childbirth because she is tied to monitoring equipment and other machines, this adds to the trauma. It is important for her to be upright and free to move about.

LOSS OF CONTROL

In a situation where control is taken away from her and she feels trapped, a survivor may relive the experience: 'Having a baby is like being abused again. I was on my back where I didn't like to be and I was out of control, and in pain.' This woman gave birth in a high-tech hospital, where she was harpooned to electronic equipment. She said that staff talked about her as if she did not exist as a person. A gaggle of student doctors stood staring at her vagina, there was a failed vacuum extraction and, finally, a forceps delivery. She felt 'like a piece of meat' and she was poked, prodded and cut. For many months afterwards she tried to come to terms with her feelings of helplessness and disempowerment. An abuse survivor may not be able to bear certain kinds of touch. One woman told me that because the midwife 'kept resting her hand on the inside of my thigh', she hit her.

A woman is much more likely to be able to control the environment and what is done to her if she has a home birth. But it is no guarantee that the experience will be positive. Sometimes midwives who have no confidence in home birth bring the hospital to the home. Often midwives receive no support from the medical system. Everything depends on the experience, personality and quality of the caregivers. Kitty had a home birth in a country where birth out of hospital is considered very abnormal, where midwives have to work in isolation from obstetricians, and where they are treated punitively if they seek to admit to hospital a client who is having a difficult birth. She told me:

I had terrible dreams, flashbacks and body memories from the birth. I still feel like my home has been violated. I couldn't birth there again, not where that happened. When I go into my bedroom I can smell blood and if my husband touches me I get flashbacks. People say it's like being sexually assaulted, but that's happened to me and this is worse. At least when I was assaulted as a kid it didn't do this kind of damage to my body. This time, there were so many people involved, and such damage, I feel like I was pack raped with a sharp instrument.

Caregivers may not be able to understand why a woman seems especially fearful, timid, passive, naive and withdrawn or, in contrast, stubborn, controlling and hostile. Though very different, compliance and confrontation are both strategies in which we try to control what is done to us when we feel attacked. Unfortunately, they usually don't work, and those in authority react with anger, defensiveness or dismissal. They may try persuasion – 'trust me' – or coercion and threats.

When birth was moved from the home to the public arena of a hospital delivery room, and turned into an industrial process with the aim of assembly-line efficiency, our technocratic culture brutalised it. A woman may be immobilised, tethered to machines and surrounded by strangers whose eyes are all apprehensively fixed on the lower end of her body. In striving to make birth safer, an intimate experience that used to take place with the support and encouragement of women friends has been transformed to an act of violence. Medical control of women's bodies turns into 'iatrogenic rape'.[84]

It is not surprising that some women prefer elective Caesarean section to vaginal birth. They hope that in this way medical gaze will be concentrated on a simple abdominal incision, they will not have to feel anything in their genitals, and the intensity of sensation vaginal labour and birth entails will be eradicated by surgery. In fact, they may surrender control over their bodies still further. Though opting for a Caesarean works for some women and can be healing, for others it is catastrophic. The abuse is re-enacted yet again. One woman decided to have a Caesarean because 'it dealt with the uncertainty. I knew exactly what was going to happen, and when. It was easier to be a body on a slab than a woman'. The surgery was badly performed, she haemorrhaged severely, the scar was slow to heal and she had massive pelvic infection. When she was pregnant again she decided she wanted a home birth, but it was difficult to organise because she was now in a high-risk category.

Even when she realises that a woman has been sexually abused, a midwife may anticipate that a woman will be co-operative if men are not involved in her care and get irritated when she proves difficult. You cannot take it for granted that simply avoiding care from men makes physical examinations easy for a survivor. If a survivor of child abuse has stored resentment against her mother because she believes she allowed abuse to continue or blamed the child for attracting sexual attention, the distrust and fear may be projected on to a female midwife or doctor. Professional caregivers represent authority and power, however personally considerate and gentle they are. An abusive father may have been kind, but 'kiss daddy good-night' was an act of exploitation disguised by soothing words and apparent tenderness. The child was betrayed.[85]

Doctors and hospital staff, however personal and friendly, are powerful because they are backed by the authority of the institution through which a woman merely passes as a patient. They receive little or no training to help them to be sensitive to this and to understand what is happening when a woman refuses to let down her defences, or when she panics during labour or at delivery as the baby's head presses against the perineum. So they ignore it, offer reassurance or give drugs for pain relief.

Pain-relieving medication does not eradicate this distress, because it is not just a matter of pain. A woman may have had an epidural and be pain-free but still feel violated. One who had been repeatedly raped by her stepfather from the age of five until she was 12, told me, 'It wasn't the pain. It was being trapped, my legs splayed out, and them doing things to me.'

In childbirth the body's usual boundaries are invaded. Caregivers take it for granted that this is so. The more intrusive the style of management the more these boundaries are attacked. A woman's genitals are exposed, she lies in the 'victim' position, while other people who are fully clothed stand around and stare at her body. She may be attached to tubes, monitors, blood pressure cuffs and other restraints. A midwife who notices that she is tense may coax her to 'relax', 'let go', perhaps 'trust your body' or 'surrender'. It is impossible for her to do this because in the past her body has betrayed her and someone in authority who was in a position of trust exploited her.

A midwife who gives 'hands off' care, and is confident and relaxed in doing so, can help the abuse survivor allow her body to work without needing to guard and defend it. A woman may feel safer in a birth pool than on a bed. The pool offers protection by providing boundaries that define the woman's own territory. There is rarely need to guard the perineum, since the warm water helps to relax tissues.[86] The midwife can watch carefully without intruding.

For a survivor, childbirth may re-awaken other anxieties about her body: 'What will the doctor discover when he examines me?' 'Are there scars? Are my labia swollen? Am I deformed?' 'Is my vagina big enough for the baby to come out?'

Paradoxically, some of the rituals designed to 'desexualise' encounters with health carers (such as avoiding eye contact) can make a woman feel depersonalised and treated like an object. To be the object of medical gaze, people staring at you as if you were a rabbit on the dissecting table, genitals exposed to a group of students – even to be observed by your partner as if your naked body were on exhibition – is likely to be distressing. One woman said, 'I have never forgiven my husband for watching me like that.' It was as if he were colluding in the violence that was being re-enacted. It can be important for a woman to state in her birth plan that students must not be present, that her body should be kept covered as far as possible, and that her partner should be at her head, sharing her view of birth, rather than staring at her bottom.

It helps to restrict the number of people coming in and out of the room and attending the birth, too. In some hospitals members of staff pop in and out without knocking. Or they knock and come straight in without waiting for permission from the woman in labour. Or they peep through a spy-hole in the door and disappear again. Staff changes contribute to this – midwives going off shift and strangers taking over. A woman may feel part of a show in which she is exhibit number one. It is much easier when there is just a midwife and partner and, perhaps, a woman birth companion.

PREPARING FOR BIRTH AFTER SEXUAL ABUSE

Giving birth is part of a woman's wider psychosexual life. It is not separate and apart from other physical experiences. This is why any survivor of abuse needs support to prepare herself emotionally for the powerful physicality of each phase of labour and birth. A woman who talked this through with her midwife said:

It was a great relief and an energising experience to be able to talk about the things I had pondered on for a long time. The midwife was very positive in reaffirming the power and ability

*that my body has to deliver. Another point that helped me feel
very powerful was that, during birth, the pain was my pain
coming from within to produce a baby.*

The pain she felt when she was abused was from that of 'being
helpless, a victim. These two kinds of pain could not be more
different. The former calls out to be felt and celebrated. The latter
demands silence, fear and shame'.[87]

Sally was expecting her first baby, a very much wanted one. She
was seven months pregnant when she plucked up courage to speak
to me about her fears. She had been sexually abused by her stepfather from when she was six until she was ten years old. She said:

*I'm terrified by how I'm going to feel when the baby's head tries
to come out. They say you feel you're going to split. That's how
it felt when he abused me. How shall I ever cope with those
terrible feelings?*

We talked about how she might respond to sensations of the baby's
head in her vagina. First there would be pressure against her anus,
then a feeling of being stretched wide, then burning like a fiery
crown round the top of a head as it slipped out. I suggested that
she could drop her jaw and let her mouth open to help her open up
below and that she could breathe, rather than push, her baby out. I
asked her how she would feel about massaging her perineum – the
tissues between her vagina and anus – with almond oil each day for
the rest of her pregnancy. I didn't want her to be under pressure to
do it, but thought it might help. She could give herself the sense of
stretching by pressing on tissues just inside her lower vulva and
spreading them apart with her finger and thumb while she consci-
entiously relaxed. She also learned how to let her pelvic floor muscles
go soft and loose, and how to tighten and hold them in a long grip
to tone them. She needed to know that this part of her body was
under her control. Sally discussed this with her partner, too. He
massaged her perineum gently as well, and helped her prepare for
the feeling of being stretched wide open.

It was good that she was having a home birth and already knew
two of the midwives and liked them. I told her that I was confident
that she would not panic and that in giving birth she could reclaim
her body from the abuse. Instead of submitting to having things
done *to* her she would use her body to give birth actively. A few
hours after her baby was born she rang:

59

It's a girl! And she's gorgeous! I didn't even tear; only a bit of bruising. I didn't rush it. I let it happen. It was wonderful! She came out bit by bit, and then when her shoulders were born the rest slid out in a whoosh. I was saying to myself, 'This is my body and this is what I want to do with it!' Now, at last, I can put the abuse behind me!

Survivors of abuse may opt for home birth because there they hope to have more control of the experience and what people do to them, and to avoid unnecessary obstetric interventions. Diane wanted a home birth because she was very frightened – 'not of the birth. I'm frightened of the medical intervention'. She had been raped when she was 14. She was worried that even though she had planned a home birth, there were eight midwives in the team and she had only met three of them. She wanted each of them to know that she didn't like being touched. After we talked she decided to tell one of the midwives whom she liked: 'She was fantastic. She said, "You're not the first."' This midwife asked Diane's permission to tell the other members about it at the group practice meeting. It was decided to have an extra on-call midwife that month so that Diane would definitely know who her midwife would be. This way Diane effectively negotiated the kind of care she wanted.

Unfortunately, it doesn't always work that way. At the antenatal clinic Zoë told her midwife that the reason why she didn't want vaginal examinations and a hospital birth was because she was sexually abused as a child. The midwife told the obstetrician, who spent two hours with Zoë trying to frighten her with the dangers of a home birth, then threatening her and concluding with an announcement that she would have to have a Caesarean. She found an independent midwife who helped her to have a home birth in water. She said: 'As a survivor of childhood sexual abuse, it was very important to have my physical integrity respected during this birth.'

Another survivor described how she worked with her midwife to make the birth of her baby a satisfying experience:

I saw the same midwife all the time ... I was not asked to undress at all ... It was understood that no one else was to enter the room unless absolutely necessary ... throughout the whole of my labour, I had no internal examinations at all. The midwife said she could tell by the length and type of contractions I was having when I entered the second stage.

A survivor of abuse may attempt to escape by mentally detaching herself from her body during childbirth. She freezes and switches off to protect herself – that was what she did when she was abused.

Distraction techniques form part of the original Lamaze training for childbirth. The simplest technique is to count aloud through a contraction. Or count objects in a visual journey around the room, or details of a pattern in fabric. Do this out loud, keeping your voice at a low pitch and deep. Don't let it become shrill. If it changes at the peak of contractions, make it a moo, not a scream.

Or use imaginative distraction, drawing on a positive visual image to recreate a scene. Use the power of your mind to lift yourself into this place. Let your uterus work like a roaring wind or crashing waves in the background. Visualise a place where you had a happy holiday, perhaps. Describe each detail – trees, hills, the scene on the beach, sea, houses, flowers – whatever you remember with pleasure, missing nothing.

This is actually a method of simple self-hypnosis in which you remain in control.

Though a distraction technique allows temporary escape, it may make it hard to reach out to your newborn baby because you feel 'on another planet'. If you can find a better way of handling the intense sensations of birth by keeping in touch with your body, vividly aware of how the baby is coming down and you are opening up, you will be right there for your baby, ready to hold your child in your arms immediately. That is a healing experience – the most healing of all.

PREGNANT AGAIN

You may have thought that you had pushed a previous distressing birth experience out of your mind. After all, months – perhaps years – have passed and the memories no longer go round and round in your head. You start another pregnancy, and then images from that birth creep in again, invading dreams and waking thoughts. What if this birth is the same?

A woman may already be several months into a pregnancy – even, perhaps, only weeks away from birth – when she starts to be tortured by intense memories that are not only mental but physical – affecting her breathing, gut, skin and muscles – and interrupting sleep.

She finds it difficult to talk to anyone else about it because they assume that she is happily expecting the new baby. If she feels like this, why did she get pregnant again? Her partner probably thought she had managed to put the distress she felt after the previous birth behind her. He would not have agreed to starting another baby if he knew they were going through all that again. She feels guilty that she should be dragging him back into the chaotic emotions that she believed she had dealt with.

She may be attending antenatal classes. She feels pity for the naiveté of women who are pregnant for the first time and who seem so hopeful and trusting. She can't mention this in discussions there. She feels terribly alone.

She needs a plan of campaign.

WAYS OF PREPARING FOR BIRTH

- Consider telling your GP or midwife, asking them to keep the information confidential. Your gut feelings about the advisability of doing this are probably your best guide.
- Ask your GP to assign you to a woman counsellor or psychotherapist. It helps if she has herself had a baby and has special understanding of sexual violence issues.
- Find out if you can be booked for one-to-one midwife care. Continuity of care from someone you know and like is important.
- Consider the option of a home birth or a birth centre.
- Be well prepared for birth by attending birth classes.
- Make a birth plan and make your priorities clear, e.g. 'No students or anyone else in the birth room other than my midwife and my partner.' 'No vaginal examinations.' 'No episiotomy without my consent.'
- If you are able to confide in your caregiver, explain why you prefer not to have vaginal examinations in pregnancy or labour. Be matter of fact about it. An experienced midwife can tell how labour is progressing by how you look and breathe.
- If you are going to have an obstetrician, consider asking for a woman, and tell her why it is important that you have only women present during your labour.
- Think about having a woman birth companion, either instead of a male partner, or to support you both. Make sure your birth companion understands the emotional support you'll need and can communicate well with your caregivers.
- Keep upright, active and moving around in labour. You do not have to be in bed or lying on your back.
- Explore a variety of ways of handling pain in childbirth. Learn about the effect – and side effects – of pain-relieving drugs.

- Also practise relaxation, slow, rhythmic breathing and 'patterned' quicker breathing as sensations become more intense. This will be useful in other stressful situations, not only birth.
- 'Letting go' may stimulate intense memories of similar letting go when you were abused. Movement may be just right for you. You don't have to lie still. Rehearse movements, especially those that involve rocking and circling your pelvis. Try these when you are upright, kneeling and on all fours.
- See if positive mental pictures help your body work more effectively. Visualisation can work well to help you 'tune in' to powerful uterine contractions. Imagine contractions as great waves that start as a ripple, build up, peak – and then ebb and stop. Or a sound image may be right for you. First you hear a single instrument – a flute or a cello, perhaps. Other instruments come in. As the contraction reaches its climax the full orchestra is playing. Then the sound begins to fade, until finally there is silence.

SOME LISTENING SKILLS

If a woman tells you she has been sexually abused, what do you say? How do you show her that you believe her and that you are an ally? How do you help her find the power within herself to cope? How can you convey that you are not making mountains out of mole hills, nor recoiling in horror, not being obtrusive, not treating her as if she was crazy, nor dismissing the experience she has been through? Penny Simkin and Phyllis Klaus draw on material from *Counselling Survivors of Childhood Sexual Abuse*[88] and expand it in their book *When Survivors Give Birth*.[89] This is how they explore a listener's possible reactions:

Non-helpful responses

- *Shock/disgust: 'Oh, my God. That's horrible. What kind of person would do such a disgusting thing to his own child?'*
- *Identification: 'How did you get through that? I don't know if I could have survived so much abuse.' Or, 'I know how you feel, because it happened to me, too.'*
- *Vicarious traumatisation: 'I feel sick just listening to your story. I can't stop thinking about it.'*

- *Anger/rage: 'Every time I hear something like that, I want to lock up every abuser and throw away the key.'*
- *Disbelief: 'Are you sure that happened? It was a long time ago and you were awfully young.'*
- *Blame: 'Why did you agree to have sex with him? Why didn't you tell your mother? Why did it go on for so long? Why didn't you make him stop or run away? Why didn't you tell someone? Why did you let him do it?'*
- *Minimising: 'Since it's all over now, and you feel you've resolved it, why don't we focus on concerns you have today?'*
- *Intrusive interest: 'What exactly did he do? How did you react? Did you respond?'*
- *Pity: 'You poor thing. You must have suffered terribly.'*
- *Rescuing: 'I'll make sure that this won't cause you any more problems.'*

The non-helpful responses such as shock, identification, or anger may be intended to be supportive by the naive counsellor, but they actually make the woman feel she's upsetting her counsellor, or that she must protect her counsellor from the truth! This demoralises the woman, adds to her shame and makes her reluctant to tell her story. Other non-helpful responses, such as disbelief, blame, minimising or intrusive interest may seem to the inexperienced counsellor as a voice of reason and perspective, but to the woman they are a realisation of her worst fear – not being believed. Such responses, or the fear of them, have silenced her in the past and will reinforce for her that no one understands or believes her. Responses such as vicarious traumatisation or rescuing indicate that the counsellor has not established appropriate boundaries.

I would add that when the listener identifies with a survivor and projects her own experience on to her she ignores the fact that though it seemed similar, it may have been a very different experience for her. When she claims that she can rescue the woman, she is taking on too much herself and disempowering her.

Helpful responses

The kind of things we say are likely to be culture-bound. They should also have an element of spontaneity and not sound practised or as if they had been read out of a book. There can be no instant made-up formulae or slick tricks. So I shall add my own observations to suggestions made by these American authors. I have worked through these responses and have suggested places where you might find that you are expressing yourself differently:

- *Calm concern: 'I'm glad you've shared your experiences with me. It's important, because sexual abuse can continue to have an impact, even in adulthood.'*
- *Acknowledge difficulty of disclosure: 'I imagine it is hard to tell me these things. It takes a lot of courage and I respect you for it.'*
- *Reinforce client's control of disclosure process: 'It can be very helpful in our work together if you can share your sexual abuse experiences since they may relate to your current concerns. However, I don't need any more detail than you are comfortable disclosing.'*
- *Acknowledge feelings: 'Sometimes when people talk about their abuse experiences it brings up very strong feelings. How are you feeling right now?'*
- *Assess well-being: 'Do you feel unsafe or fearful in any aspect of your life?'*

The helpful responses reassure the woman that her counsellor can handle her story and that the woman has a strong and capable ally in her healing process.

It may help if you go through these responses, putting them in your own words. Then reflect on what you have said in the past. Have you been tempted to say some of the things that are listed under 'Non-helpful responses' (see pp. 63–4)? Now think how you might express yourself in future. Maybe the language of these responses sounded rather formal to you. Do you want to adapt it so that you are using more everyday speech? Remember, too, that when we are in conversation we don't always use full and grammatical sentences. Sometimes a phrase or a word is better:

- Would you say 'adulthood' and 'have an impact'?
- This is an American way of assuring the survivor that she is in control. Think of alternatives to 'relate to your current concerns' and 'comfortable disclosing'. Perhaps change this to 'Since they may be connected with your fears about birth. But I don't need to know anything more than you want to tell me.'

- Again, what might you say in place of the last sentence? 'How does it feel at the moment?'
- You could put this more casually: 'Are there times in life when you don't feel safe or get very afraid?'

THE CHILDBIRTH EDUCATOR

It is best to assume that there are survivors in any group you are teaching. You don't have to know for sure. You certainly should not single out victims. The kind of preparation for birth that is right for a survivor of sexual abuse is right for everyone else in the class, too. It provides a good standard for antenatal teaching. It is likely that every childbirth class has at least one survivor of child abuse. You may feel vaguely uncomfortable about a woman whom you don't realise has been sexually abused but who is especially timid and compliant or, on the contrary, is in a constant 'yes, but' mode. These are elements in survival strategy. A woman may be submissive, thinking that, if she is not, she will somehow be punished. Or she challenges whatever you say, or reacts with stubborn scepticism. This can prove irritating, and you may not understand why you can't form a positive relationship with her and why she responds with hostility. Some abuse survivors are reluctant to make a birth plan because they want to avoid conflict. Others produce a rigid plan, which you know will cause conflict. You cannot conclude that a woman has experienced sexual abuse because she is definite about what she wants, on the one hand, or is reluctant to 'make a fuss', on the other. Be careful not to medicalise or to stereotype ways in which women in the class think and behave.

The teacher's task is to empower everyone in the class. An important element in this is negotiating the kind of care they want. For different women this will be a home birth, an epidural or an elective Caesarean section. It often helps to involve members of the class in research – getting more information about the effects and side effects of medical practices and conditions in different hospitals in the area. This will add to their understanding and knowledge and increase self-confidence.

In classes, the language you use should always be inclusive, accepting in a matter-of-fact way that some women in the group will have been sexually abused and/or disempowered. An abuse survivor does not want to be labelled. Always give 'we' messages instead of 'you' messages.

Do not assume, however, that everyone who has been abused will be especially vulnerable. The opposite may be true. Coping with that experience may have enabled a woman to draw on her inner strength. She brings emotional strength and resilience to childbirth.

One risk a woman runs with disclosing to caregivers that she was sexually abused as a child is that all her wishes and actions may be pathologised and accounted for entirely in terms of the abuse. When a woman states that she does not want vaginal examinations or would like to be upright and free to move, rather than lying supine, it should *not* be explained by reference to previous sexual abuse. Every woman should be able to say what she wants, and be supported by a midwife in doing so. If she has made a detailed birth plan, this is not a sign that she has been sexually abused. Previous experiences of medical treatment may have had this effect. Or she may simply be an assertive woman who tackles life challenges in that way.

THE PARTNER

- Discuss her priorities about how people care for her and the atmosphere in the room.
- Create a safe space for her.
- Follow her lead. Because you know her well and may have had to negotiate how and where she wants to be touched in love making, you know what is likely to stimulate memories of the abuse and what is likely to help her.
- Give her strong backing in pregnancy and birth so that *she* makes the decisions, not the professionals.
- When a course of action is suggested that entails an intervention, say that you want to consider this together. You need a short time in private to talk about it.

THE DOULA

- A doula or other female birth companion can give strong support to anyone who has experienced sexual abuse.
- Sometimes there are difficulties.
- A client may be heavily dependent on the doula to protect her against professional caregivers whom she distrusts.

67

- An important part of a birth companion's task is to foster good communication, but she may get caught in the middle and feel trapped between them.
- It is important to talk through with her client ahead of time her priorities, her hopes and fears, the kind of atmosphere she wants created in the birth room, and ways in which they can work together to achieve this.

HOW A MIDWIFE CAN HELP A WOMAN WHO HAS BEEN SEXUALLY ABUSED

In pregnancy

- Never assume that a woman has been abused, and if a client tells you that she has, do not think of her as a special 'case', or that you now know everything you need to know about her.
- Give time to listen and listen reflectively. Do not make judgements. Arrange one-to-one care for her so that she never has to deal with strangers.
- Discuss a range of options about the place of birth. Give her the information and make sure she is free to decide whatever she feels is best.
- Protect her against medical gaze. Ensure that she has privacy. Keep intruders out of the room.
- Ask for her consent before touching her.
- Ask a more general question, too. 'Do you have any no-go areas?'
- Communicate well with her partner and any other birth companion. Any form of conflict, even though hidden, pollutes the birth environment. Work together to create an atmosphere of confidence and tranquillity.
- Draw on your own inner resources of strength and energy. Keep focused. Do not let what you have to give of yourself be dissipated in busyness.
- See if you can arrange for antenatal care to be given in a woman's own territory – her home – rather than in the official territory of a clinic or hospital.
- Explain the purpose of each test and examination before you do it. Tell her what it will involve, how long it will last, and where exactly she will be touched. Do this while she is sitting

clothed, so that she becomes a colleague in finding out answers to questions, rather than a subject you screen.

In childbirth

- Ask the woman in advance what words and phrases will encourage and relax her. Practise a few. Does she want to be touched, or not? If so, how and where? Might massage help or not? Practise this, too, and see how it works. Are there any particular words that might be harmful? What kind of touch, and where, must you avoid? The important thing is to let her guide you.
- Do not take over. Do not manage her. Do not dominate. She should be able to control what you do, and be fully supported in this. If she feels swept away by the power of labour, ask her if she wants you to take charge for a while, discuss how, and follow her instructions. This is most likely to happen when she is in transition between the first and second stages and contractions are coming almost continuously.
- When you think that she will soon want to push, tell her, so that she is prepared for it. But do not get her pushing on command. Let her know that everything is going well and that there is no hurry. Her body will tell her the right time for pushing.

69

The birth experiences of women who have been sexually abused throw light on the power dynamics of any medical encounter and the inequalities between the givers and receivers of care. The experiences of women who have been sexually abused represent in microcosm those of all women who feel degraded and abused by what is done to them in pregnancy and childbirth.

When birth is conducted with no personal consideration and respect, when management is crude and insensitive, it is itself a form of sexual abuse.

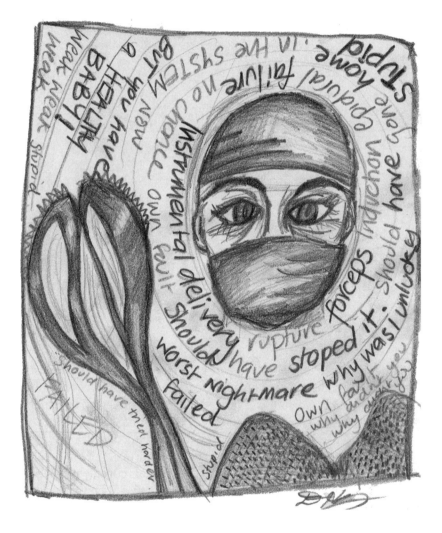

FLASHBACKS, PANIC ATTACKS AND NIGHTMARES

6

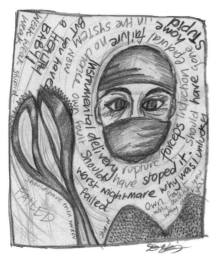

FLASHBACKS ARE NOT JUST VIDID MEMORIES. They are not only in the mind. They are intense physical replays of distressing experiences that involve breathing, muscles, heart rate, galvanic skin response and gut. A woman may turn white, get goose pimples and be unable to speak. Her eyes are fixed. She becomes suddenly paralysed. The word that a woman sometimes uses to describe her feelings during the birth experience itself is 'petrified'. When she relives it she is frozen into immobility again. She gasps, chokes or screams, may lose control of bladder or bowels or vomit. Her hair stands on end, and she may faint. A flashback is often stimulated by, and in turn affects, sight, hearing, smell, taste and touch.

FLASHBACKS

One woman experienced flashbacks when she smelt curry. The midwives had been snatching a takeaway while she was in a traumatic labour. For another it was the odour of the disinfectant used in the maternity unit. A woman almost fainted when she took her baby to the GP to be immunised and saw the needle about to penetrate the skin. Another, who said that childbirth had been like torture, was at a church service and noticed a very pregnant woman. In an instant she 'became' that woman with a foreboding of pain and doom and had a flashback. A flashback may strike when a woman watches TV and sees someone in a sitcom go into labour or deliver a baby, even when this is intended to be comedy.

Many women say that they cannot go in to the hospital to visit a friend, or even walk past it, because of flashbacks:

> *The birth of my baby was horrendous. I feel I was violated. I can't face going back to the hospital to talk to anyone there about it. I can't even drive past the hospital without breaking out into a sweat . . . I have nightmares and flashbacks to the birth, as if it were happening all over again. I feel I haven't any control over anything.*

The unexpected sight of someone who was present during the traumatic experience – a doctor or one of the midwives, for example – may trigger a flashback; even, occasionally, a woman's own partner seen from a particular angle may do this. One woman has to avoid lying on her back at night, and during sex, because then she has flashbacks to when she lay helpless, unable to move after an epidural, while 'the doctor pushed his fingers up my vagina, telling me to trust him and asking if I could feel it. I felt raped'.

A woman who gave birth on bonfire night said that fireworks were going off during her labour and now the sound of exploding brings immediate flashbacks. Any situation in which a woman's body is being probed may trigger them, as it did for one who had an emergency Caesarean and experienced a flashback at the dentist and again when she had a coil fitted.

Five months after a Caesarean section that terminated a long and painful labour in which she 'failed to progress', a woman went to her dentist to have a bridge put in:

> *I remember sitting down very reclined, the light very bright above my face and the dentist wearing a mask. He started putting a clay*

mould to take the shape of my teeth and he was pressing down my mouth. Suddenly my heart started going fast, my blood went to my head, I needed air to breathe and my arms were starting to lift. [I was in tears and] wanted to run as far as I could. The dentist and the nurse stopped doing what they were doing and got very worried and puzzled without understanding what on earth was going on with their patient. I was re-experiencing what happened to me in theatre.

Another woman described her flashbacks this way:

They put me up in the stirrups and everything and I kept trying to close my legs, and they kept opening my legs up, and they're touching me and wiping me. You can feel them pulling and pushing at you, and I kept pushing them away.

This woman also had nightmares in which she was suing someone for raping her.

Sex triggers flashbacks, too, especially when a woman lies on her back, legs raised and apart as if being examined in lithotomy (lying on her back with her legs parted, supported by long stirrups and knees wide apart) or having an instrumental delivery. A woman whose obstetrician held the forceps up to show her 'and clanged them together' told me, 'I remember screaming inside, but on the outside watching it and being unable to do anything. I remember watching her put the forceps in and it makes me physically sick to think about it.' When she has sex she tries to feel nothing – she says: 'I have to concentrate hard on not seeing the forceps.'

Flashbacks may occur when a woman is 'off guard', waking from sleep in the morning or relaxing during the day. This makes her frightened to take any rest and fuels the frenetic activity that is a common feature of PTSD.

The essence of a flashback is that it is uncontrollable. You cannot get rid of it with mind power, distract yourself, pretend it is not there or reason yourself out of it. It takes over and disempowers you.

PANIC ATTACKS

Panic attacks also take place without warning, even without a clear flashback. A mother is convinced that something dreadful has happened to her baby or other child. She can't face meeting someone or going into a crowded room, and sometimes is unable to leave

73

the house. She may be locked into immobility and rigid with fear. During a panic attack she sweats and her skin feels cold and clammy. She can feel her heart pound and there is a drumming in her ears. She may gasp and hyperventilate, breathing heavily and rapidly, flushing out carbon dioxide from her bloodstream so that the natural balance of blood gases is lost. This makes her light-headed and giddy, and can even result in fainting. One woman who had a previous traumatic birth told me how she felt during her next (unplanned) pregnancy:

> *I tried to be very strong and never let anyone know that it bothered me, but I would often late at night just curl up in a ball in bed, bury my head in a pillow and cry and cry. Going back to the hospital was very very hard. I had to have a scan. I thought, 'It can't be that bad – no prob!' But on the way there in the car I was in floods of tears. I was nearly late as I was trying to gain some sort of composure before going in.*

Anyone who suspects that a woman is having a flashback or panic attack should avoid reaching out to hold her. This is likely to make her feel more trapped, and perhaps attacked. It is important not to panic yourself, but to 'hold' and 'contain' her distress, and to be there for her after the crisis is passed, acknowledging rather than ignoring it, accepting it as an experience that is painfully intense, but can be dealt with.

There is little understanding by some caregivers of the uncontrollable horror of panic attacks. A woman who had two traumatic births was admitted to hospital at 29 weeks for a planned Caesarean because of placenta praevia. The claustrophobia and panic attacks she experienced were so severe that she ran out of the hospital in her pyjamas. The hospital manager was called in. He reprimanded her, 'You've got to do things our way. You're either here doing as we tell you, or we can't do anything for you.' One of the midwives complained, 'You've spoilt my day!' Both appeared to have no comprehension of her distress and her need for understanding.

NIGHTMARES

A woman may be unable to let herself drift into sleep because of nightmares. She lies in bed willing herself to relax and let go, but cannot. The dreams that break into her sleep are too horrific. One painted me a picture of a recurrent nightmare in which she lay supine and naked on a delivery table, unable to move or show her distress because of drugs she had received prior to surgery, with doctors and nurses standing over her wearing leering devil masks, the baby separated from her inside a glass bottle. It expressed the helplessness and terror she felt as she had a Caesarean section, and her isolation from the child who had been cut out of her. Another woman described repeated dreams of experiments on young Jewish girls at the hands of the Nazis and 'Shining Path' types of atrocities. She said:

I have nightly dreams about a large range of unfortunate events. I don't like to be in bed long. I get up out of bed on average three times per night. I generally sleep between four or five hours altogether. I tend to wake frightened.

She had an episiotomy, performed before the numbing injection had time to take effect, that cut into her rectum. Another woman, with an episiotomy that extended in a laceration, said she lay in bed 'and the whole story would go round and round in my head. I would have dreams where I was strapped back down being stitched up with all those people looking, and screaming and screaming and no one would listen'. Another told me, 'For three months after my daughter was born every night when I closed my eyes to go asleep I had flashbacks.'

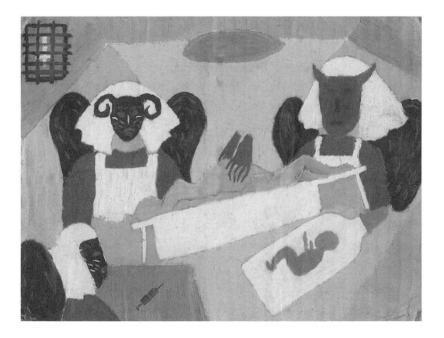

A woman who is on red alert is hyper-vigilant, watching her baby for signs of abnormality and illness like a hawk. Being on constant alert and sleeping spasmodically leads to exhaustion. She may be startled at any unexpected touch, sound or other intrusion. She feels both tense and drained. She cannot concentrate, and may get very irritable with those nearest to her. At the same time she feels isolated from everyone around her, imprisoned in her own shell. She fears she is going insane.

No amount of coaxing a woman to relax, counselling her not to dwell on what happened during the birth or telling her to focus on her lovely baby will counteract post-traumatic stress following a distressing birth. Above all, she needs her experience validated, both how she felt then and how she feels now. She needs someone who will stand beside her and help her face it, instead of trying to run away from, trivialise and ignore the pain.

Flashbacks, nightmares and panic attacks are symptoms that lead to a diagnosis of PTSD as defined by the American Psychiatric Association in its *Diagnostic and Statistical Manual*.[90] This is a reality, not something imagined by a woman who just can't pull herself together and wants a psychiatric label to justify poor performance as a mother. Though having a medical tag may not appear to be life enhancing, many women breathe a sigh of relief when at last their emotional pain can be given a name.

Post-traumatic stress is not a mental illness, however. It is 'a normal response to an abnormal event rather than a pathological condition'.[91]

There is some evidence of chemical changes in the brain of anyone who is suffering from PTSD, chemicals that control coping behaviour, learning and memory. Brain imaging studies record altered metabolism and blood flow.[92] Someone with PTSD is likely to have abnormal levels of hormones stimulated by stress. Cortisol levels are below normal and epinephrine and norepinephrine higher. Thyroid function may be altered, as is the transmission of serotonin and opiates between nerves. When we are aware of danger, natural opiates that reduce pain are triggered in the bloodstream. People who suffer from PTSD continue to produce these high levels after the threat has passed.

It was once believed that anybody who could carry on as normal after trauma was responding in a 'healthy' way. We know now that this is not true. A 'stiff upper lip' can be dangerous.

- Recurring and intrusive recollections of an unexpected and threatening event that anyone would agree was distressing.
- Having nightmares about it.
- Flashbacks: suddenly feeling that it is happening again, often with hallucinations and illusions.
- Distress when anything occurs that reminds you of what happens, or symbolises it – your baby's birthday, for example. When birth comes up in discussion, or another woman describes her birth – even a happy one – you go numb.
- You try to escape feelings that stem from the trauma. It is normal to avoid any activities or situations that remind you of it, so you pull away from social encounters that entail meeting pregnant women and new mothers, for example. You don't switch on the TV if there is anything on to do with pregnancy or birth. It is difficult to reach out, feel and respond to other people's feelings and this may include those of your baby. You detach yourself and are emotionally numb.
- You may not remember many things about the labour and birth. This has a name: 'psychogenic amnesia'. Memories are fragmented, like a jigsaw puzzle that has been thrown on the floor and scattered. You only recognise disconnected bits of it. Even when your partner or a caregiver explains what happened – expecting you to accept the reality of what they are describing and why it happened – and goes through the case notes, it does not make sense. You may nod and agree in order to silence them. You are grateful that they bother, but what they say does not match your personal experience. It is another order of reality.

A woman may not remember signing a consent form for a Caesarean, or that a particular individual came into the room, or that she was involved in any discussion about interventions that took place. She may not remember seeing and holding her baby. Her version of events is quite different from the official version.

This is one reason why routine debriefing after a traumatic birth is rarely enough. Sometimes it does more harm than good, since it may present a birth account that is dramatically opposed to the woman's own experience, and appear to her to be a confidence trick and an attempt at brainwashing. Birth Afterthoughts and similar projects where a midwife goes through a woman's notes with her can seem like efforts to silence her, masquerading as sympathy and understanding.

She may be right. Hospital managers want to prevent complaints, avoid official investigations and keep the system running smoothly. Birth Afterthoughts schemes are often justified because they reduce the number of complaints from patients and make it less likely that the hospital will be sued.

One woman who rang me after a Caesarean in which the obstetrician had sliced open her baby's cheek with a scalpel by mistake, said the Birth Afterthoughts midwife glanced at the baby and remarked, 'Oh, it's hardly noticeable!', as if she was making a fuss about nothing. In fact, the wound was infected and seven months later there was still an obvious scar. The obstetrician had apologised, but said she 'didn't know he was there'. There was no mention of the injury in the record of the birth.

Case records are sometimes incomplete, with entries written in after the event. Occasionally, items are deleted and others added that misrepresent what occurred to prevent the hospital or members of staff being sued.

Medical records need to be approached with a healthy scepticism, especially when there are obvious alterations and omissions. Never seek reality from case notes.

On the other hand, going through the official record of a labour with someone who is not on the defensive, who takes time to explain and who listens to you can be part of the process of healing. The midwife who comes to see you is likely to be genuinely concerned to help you to start to get together at least some pieces of the jigsaw and see parts of the picture. You do not have to agree with everything that is described. And it may be that no one is deliberately trying to mislead you or explain away the horrific events that occurred.

There is no compulsion to trust anybody. Just listen and learn. If you have a birth partner with you, go through the notes together and photocopy them to discuss later. Explore them afterwards without feeling under pressure, and in your own time.

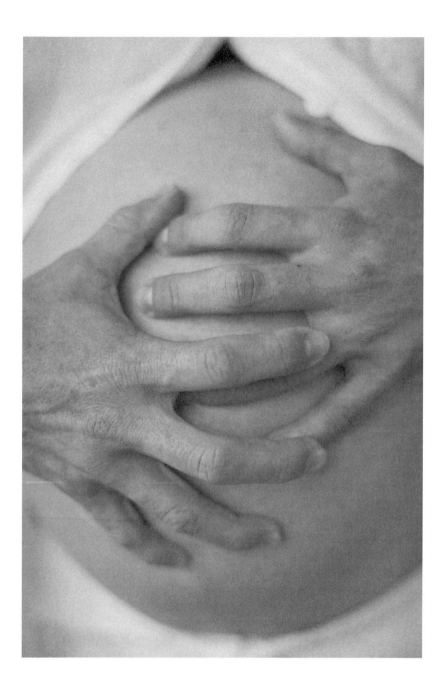

PAIN

7

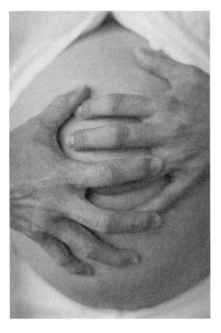

WHEN A WOMAN STARTS TO TALK about her traumatic birth she often describes the experience in terms of pain. That word is a flag with which she signals the need to have distress acknowledged and understood. Yet as her narrative unfolds, the single concept 'pain' becomes much more complex. It emerges that it was pain she could not manage or control because of what other people were doing to her. It was pain with which she was trapped.

Human beings have an almost identical threshold of sensation for pain. The idea of 'high' and 'low' pain thresholds is false. In lab experiments with electric shocks people report a pain sensation at the same point. But pain is never just a sensation. Everything that is going on in our brains – cognitive processes – including the type of attention we give to the sensation, affect the way we feel pain. This in turn is modified by the environment, the social context of the pain experience. We can be too busy to focus on pain. When we feel nurtured and protected pain has a different quality from when we feel vulnerable. If it is suggested that pain is dangerous and destructive the sensation is different from a setting in which it is perceived as positive and creative and a sign that our bodies are doing good work. When our attention is entirely directed to the pain sensation it is harder to tolerate than if attention is focused on a desired outcome.

If we are stressed, fearful and anxious, a pain sensation that we can handle well when we are relaxed and happy may overwhelm us. If we anticipate that pain will be severe, it makes it more likely, because we are already tense and alarmed, in a state of fight or flight. When we feel we cannot control the stimulus, pain is worse than when we have ways of controlling it. Even a strong drug such as morphine does not work as well – and may even not work at all – if anxiety is raised to a high level.

If we are active, the sensation of pain may become incidental – a side effect of the activity in which we are engaged, rather than dominating us. This is why athletes, footballers and mountain climbers may not notice pain that in other circumstances would be overwhelming. Feeling out of control and roller-coasted by decisions made by other people can make even a straightforward labour traumatic.[93]

Pain is hardest to bear when it hits suddenly, instead of building up slowly. This is one reason why induction and artificial stimulation of labour can produce overwhelming pain. These interventions trigger stress because the shock that comes from the pain demonstrates that we cannot cope, and raises alarm signals about the future. If it is this bad now, at the beginning of labour, what is it going to be like in an hour's time – and longer?

Pain is distinct from what has been called 'fitness'. A woman may have a painful labour that she still finds 'satisfying'. That word is often used in birth research and is difficult to define. It is not just a passive feeling, 'Oh, it was all right'. Maybe 'fulfilment' describes it better, though that, too, is a passive term that does nothing to suggest the gusto and exhilaration that a woman may experience in birth, in spite of pain. Recent research attempts to measure 'fitness'. It is partly to do with physical strength, which is affected by tiredness, hypoglycaemia and exhaustion. But it is also linked to psychological strength: motivation, involvement and 'some inner strength to go through the experience of childbirth'.[94]

There is evidence to show that in childbirth pain is hardest to bear when other things happen that put a woman under stress. These have been well described as 'noxious stimuli'.[95] Pain is accentuated when labour is managed actively, leading to an avalanche of interventions when movement is restricted. This is especially the case when a woman is confined to bed, when there is a policy of nil by mouth (especially when fluids are restricted), when an intravenous infusion is set up, or when there are continuous electronic fetal monitoring and/or routine cervical exams. The hospital environment contributes to this when there is no privacy, when strangers intrude and when the surroundings are uncomfortable, with bright lights and noise. An almost certain way of ensuring that a woman has intolerable pain is to deny her continuous personal support through labour and birth.

KILLING PAIN WITH DRUGS

Anaesthesia to abolish the pain of birth was first introduced by James Simpson in the nineteenth century. Queen Victoria was a strong advocate of chloroform because she used it herself and thought it was wonderful. In the United States famous obstetricians such as Walter Channing of Harvard, and later J. Whitridge Williams and Joseph DeLee, were powerful advocates of obstetric anaesthesia. Fear of childbirth began to be discussed in articles in women's magazines. Those who anticipated that they would be unconscious at delivery had been conditioned by doctors to believe that the birth of the baby's head was agonising. They were usually left to cope with the pain of the labour themselves. Williams wrote:

As soon as the head begins to distend the vulva, the patient's sufferings become greatly increased, and are frequently excruciating. If anaesthesia has not already been induced, its use should be begun at this stage, partly to relieve the pain, and partly to aid in protecting the perineum.[96]

The result was that women missed out on the most exultant part of birth – the baby slipping out. They were heavily anaesthetised and often came to only when the baby was washed and dressed and shown to them. A medical sociologist writes:

For at least 70 years beginning in the 1890s, physicians did not anesthetize women during transition, the most painful portion of labor. Rather, they rendered women unconscious at the moment of birth. Physicians based this therapeutically useless but long sacrosanct medical practise on what they presumed women felt, given the disturbing way women looked at the moment of birth. Women accepted this practise because they were ignorant of the sensations of birth. Thus physicians' and women's perceptions of labor pain, rather than reality, have played a major historic role in shaping the administration of obstetric anaesthesia.[97]

Because women believed what they were told by obstetricians, they campaigned strongly for twilight sleep, a mixture of scopolamine and morphine that produced a state of semi-consciousness, in which the woman felt pain, but could not remember it. Patients who had been 'scoped' were caged in high-barred, padded cots to prevent injuries when they flung themselves around in manic frenzy.

A GOOD BIRTH

There is a strong association between women having positive birth experiences and feeling that they are in control. This includes being in control of what caregivers do to them, in control of how they themselves behave in labour and in control during contractions. It is difficult for most women to feel that they have any control over the way birth is managed. A study of control in childbirth analysed data from 1,146 women, of whom 39.5 per cent felt they could control what was done to them, whereas 61 per cent felt in control of their own behaviour.[98] Women who had given birth before were much more likely to feel they had control over what was done to them, as well as their own behaviour, and also over pain. It is usually claimed that second births are easier, but it is probably not just a matter of physiology: the second time round a woman is well rehearsed.

But this doesn't always happen. As we have seen already, some women have a positive first birth and then go on to have a bad experience with the next one. Lynette had her first baby in France in a small birth centre with midwives she knew. Then she had the next one in a large London hospital where she felt alternately neglected and bullied; the labour was distressing and painful, and she suffered post-traumatic stress afterwards.

Women are often told that bad birth memories will fade and they will not remember the pain. But women do not 'forget' the experience of birth. They remember it, and over the following months it may get worse as they look back on it. A Swedish study reveals that 47 per cent of women make the same assessment of pain intensity one year after birth as they did two months post-partum, and 60 per cent assess the total experience in the same way as they did 10 months before.[99] However, there is wide variation in recall of pain and the total birth experience, and this varies with time. It should not be taken for granted that if women feel positive about birth at two months post-partum they will feel equally positive 10 months later. They often express relief and euphoria just after birth, but are unhappy about the experience later in the first year.

ENTONOX AND OPIATES

Gas and oxygen (Entonox) – a mix of oxygen and nitrous oxide – is the mildest form of pain-relieving drug available and does not affect the baby, because every time the mother breathes out the drug is removed from her bloodstream. It is inhaled through a mouthpiece or mask and is under the control of the woman herself. It is important to start breathing in the gas as the contraction begins, and not wait until pain is felt. It takes the edge off contractions.

The disadvantages of opiate drugs are well documented and have been known for many years.[100] They may affect the baby because they are central nervous system depressants. As a result, the baby is likely to have a low Apgar score and may not breathe well at birth.[101] A systematic review of 48 studies of the effects of opioids did not examine whether or not they affected breastfeeding or bonding.[102] But some studies have examined newborn behaviour after the mother has had opioids and revealed a significant effect. The baby may be drowsy and unresponsive and fail to root for the breast or suckle.[103]

A newborn baby who has not been exposed to analgesia behaves differently from one who has. For example, without drugs most babies share what has been called 'inborn pre-feeding behaviour'. Twenty-eight newborn babies were filmed on video after they had been dried and placed between their mothers' naked breasts straight after birth. These videos were analysed blindly (i.e. the researchers did not know which mothers had had drugs for pain relief). There were three groups of women. One group had had no analgesia. One had had mepaivicaine in a pudendal block and another either pethidine or bupaivicaine, or more than one type of analgesia. Only half the babies of mothers who had received drugs breastfed in the first two and a half hours after birth. All the babies of mothers who had no analgesia breastfed. The babies in the analgesia group were less likely to stroke and massage their mothers' breasts, make hand to mouth movements, touch the nipple with their hands, lick it and suckle.[104] They also had higher temperatures and cried more. Researchers concluded that 'several types of analgesia given to the mother during labor may interfere with a newborn's spontaneous breast-seeking and breastfeeding behaviors and increase the new-born's temperature and crying.'

It is often claimed that epidurals have no effect on the baby at all. But after an epidural babies score worse on the Brazelton Neonatal Behavioral Assessment scale.[105] Women may choose an epidural when labour is induced because they realise that there is likely to be more pain. Fifty-six per cent of women in the UK did so in the year 2002–3, compared with 12 per cent of those for whom labour started spontaneously.[106]

When a woman who hoped to handle birth without painkilling drugs cannot cope with the pain, she often feels guilty that she 'gave in'. Sometimes midwives seem to her to take it as a sign that at last she is being reasonable and accepting their superior knowledge about birth pain. She *submits* to analgesia. It can seem like a triumph of the system over a woman who was bravely resisting. There is a sense of humiliation and defeat.

With her self-confidence destroyed, she surrenders control of the labour. Medication for pain relief is preceded or followed by contin-uous electronic fetal monitoring, immobilisation, artificial uterine stimulation and more medication, and this is likely to lead to concern about the fetal heart rate and an assisted delivery or crash Caesarean section. When all this happens, a woman often feels that she has been very silly in thinking that she could cope with labour without drugs.

Given the possible side effects of pain-relieving drugs, it is entirely reasonable to aim to go through labour without medication. Opiates, such as pethidine, have the effect of 'detaching' the mother from pain and tranquillising her. But the relaxation that results is more like that of a drunk staggering along the road than that of a yogi deep in concentration. One woman told me, 'I felt a zombie.' Another said, 'The midwife gave me an injection. I found out from my notes that it was a large dose of morphine, and I was unconscious pretty much from then on.' She could neither talk nor move. 'The morphine just trapped me in a world of pain, unable to help myself.' A typical sequence of events is described in an account from a woman who tells what happens after there was a shift change. A 'bossy midwife' took over from a 'lovely' one who had supported her constantly so that she felt she was 'coping very well' and had had her labouring in a warm bath. The new midwife 'decided I needed to be monitored':

> *I was strapped to the monitor and left alone. The pain was getting really bad and she suggested I have a pethidine injection. I agreed and she sounded so confident it would help. It didn't, I was in the same amount of pain, except I felt like I'd had way too much to drink. I couldn't even talk properly and had to crawl to go to the toilet. I started to panic, then my labour stopped. The midwife said she would have to break my waters and set up a drip to induce the contractions. I was still falling around the place drunk, I hadn't slept in two nights and had had nothing to eat or drink. The contractions were hitting me like a ton of bricks and I was in unbelievable agony, stuck on my back with all the drips and monitors. I then had an epidural. It must have worked for a bit as I fell asleep for an hour or two. When I woke up it was only working on one side and I was in agony again. When it came to the delivery I was given about two chances to push, and the midwife said 'I'm going to have to cut you' and I was screaming at her not to do it, but she did it anyway. I felt so exhausted and couldn't even hold the baby. I felt nothing and I just wanted to sleep. The baby was taken away.*

Drugged with opiates, a woman may lose all control: her speech is slurred, she giggles or weeps, she is without purpose and direction, and incapable of rational thought. She feels sick and may vomit.[107] The fetal heart slows.[108,109] As contractions get more powerful, with all her defences down, the pain can be overwhelming. At this point she is likely to be offered an epidural.

THE EPIDURAL

An epidural is often suggested when a woman feels at her most vulnerable. It may seem to be the solution for someone who cannot bear to see her in pain. Even so, she may have to wait for it because the anaesthetist is not available. Women report waiting an hour, and sometimes longer.

An epidural is often used in place of emotional support. A midwife may be trying to attend two or three women at the same time and cannot give one-to-one care. A woman told me she felt very isolated in labour, 'not getting any positive feedback on how well I was doing. I only remember the midwife sitting and writing notes'. She was examined after several hours and found to be still only 3 centimetres dilated. The midwife told her, 'Nothing has changed.' Her partner mentioned an epidural. 'The epidural was going to fix it – for him. From that point on I felt everything running away with me. Dazed and confused – compliant. I don't remember feeling pain. I felt totally numb and tired.'

Moreover, once an epidural is given, support may be withdrawn – even if it was previously available – because a midwife is busy and the mother is clearly not in pain.

An epidural is highly effective at killing pain. Nowadays it can often be given so that the mother still feels touch and feels her baby emerging from her vagina. But it has side effects. Because her blood pressure may drop, oxygen flowing to her baby is reduced and its heart slows down or beats abnormally fast.[110,111] Since she cannot pass urine, a catheter is inserted. Her temperature rises – resulting in the fetal temperature rising, too. Moreover, contractions may get weaker so that she is then given oxytocin to augment labour. An epidural adds, on average, an hour to a labour. The pushing stage is likely to be extended. This in turn is likely to lead to an instrumental delivery or possibly to Caesarean section because the baby is in a difficult position, though it is difficult to isolate cause and effect.[112,113,114] The risk of a severe perineal tear is increased with an instrumental delivery.

When an epidural is still effective in the second stage the mother will be pushing without any physical sensations to guide her. Relying entirely on instructions, pushing is co-ordinated with peaks of contractions. It is rather as if she is trying to swallow but cannot feel the food in her mouth, or is throwing a ball when her hand and arm are numb.

The anaesthetic may have slackened usually springy pelvic floor muscles, too. They sag like the over-stretched sleeve of a jersey. Though this sounds a good thing – as it might allow more space for the baby to get out – if the pelvic floor has lost its tone, when the baby's head descends on to these muscles it may not rotate to the perfect angle for birth and the head may stick in the transverse position. Or it may start to turn and get stuck. This is deep transverse arrest, a condition that calls for delivery by ventouse or forceps. There is reduced risk of needing an instrumental delivery if a woman has a low-dose 'mobile' epidural.[115,116]

If a woman has had an epidural and has no spontaneous urge to push, it is best not to push until the head can be seen on the perineum. The birth being delayed is another reason for delivery having to be assisted by forceps or vacuum extraction. There are obstetricians, however, who assert that a woman should push immediately she is fully dilated, because 'delayed pushing blocks labour ward beds unnecessarily'.[117] This is not for the benefit of the mothers but for efficient crowd control and management of the hospital.

Many women become exhausted with prolonged breath-holding and straining. They get dehydrated, too. They hyperventilate, and ketones appear in their urine from burning up fat. Blood vessels burst in their eyes and faces. They are drenched with sweat, and after the birth they have a sore throat and their muscles ache as if they have flu.

Some women have only partial pain relief from an epidural. It may be one-sided. This lop-sided pain can be even more difficult to handle than pain that is felt as a circular muscular squeeze.

If the drug is not inserted correctly, punctures the dura and enters the spinal cavity, there will be leakage of spinal fluid. This is called a 'spinal tap'. The mother gets a severe headache and has to lie completely flat. It can be treated with a blood patch, her own blood being injected to seal the leak. Even so, occasionally the spinal headache lasts for weeks, or even months.

Sometimes an epidural does not work at all. An obstetrician performing an instrumental delivery may not realise that the patient can feel everything and goes ahead with an episiotomy and forceps extraction. A doctor may suture the perineum without realising that it is not anaesthetised:

> *I was stitched by a student and I had a room full of people. I was so out of it I couldn't even say anything. [She had pethidine before the epidural.] I was given no anaesthetic and the stitching, as it was a cut going into a tear, took 30 minutes. The student kept making mistakes and was having to take stitches out and do them again. All I could do was lay there and wait for it to be over.*

When a baby's temperature has been raised by an epidural, the mother and baby often have investigations for infection and are dosed with antibiotics just in case. Another side effect is that some women who have epidurals experience bladder numbness afterwards and must have a catheter inserted for 24–48 hours; some have long-term bladder dysfunction or faecal incontinence.[118,119]

An epidural – even one that effectively relieves pain and has few side effects – is no guarantee that birth is a satisfying experience. A longitudinal Swedish study of 2,541 women that measured their experience of labour and birth one year later concluded:

> Women's request for an epidural block should always be respected, but . . . pain relief did not necessarily improve women's experience of childbirth. Such a request may also indicate a need for emotional support. [This] may be a more effective way for women to cope with labor than obstetric analgesia.[120]

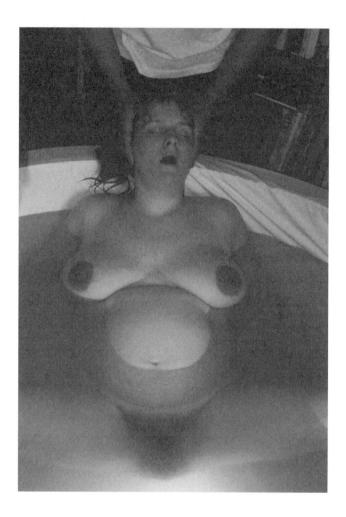

OTHER WAYS OF
HANDLING PAIN

8

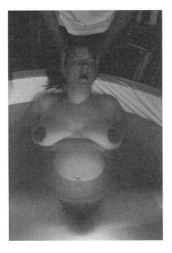

Y OU MAY BE LOOKING FOR OTHER WAYS of handling pain – ones
you can control yourself, and which have few or no side effects
for both you and your baby.

A pregnant woman who is approaching birth dreading the pain
and fearful that she will not be able to cope with it needs to explore
her options. It is not a question of just choosing between drugs. She
can also consider ways of handling pain herself or with the help of
a birth partner or a specialist in alternative ways of dealing with
pain. *She* is in control – not the professionals.

Strong emotional support and comfort given by someone who can be relied on to be present without fail whenever needed makes an astonishing difference.

The most effective way of handling pain without drugs is nothing to do with techniques or training, and does not involve learning a new skill or esoteric mental or physical activity. It is simply having another woman with you to give constant, unstinting support and who, because she has confidence in you, instils the self-confidence that yes, you can really do this; you can give birth.

A BIRTH COMPANION

Fourteen randomised controlled trials show that women who have continuous one-to-one support are less likely to use drugs for pain relief.[121] This person should be with the mother right through labour, should respond sensitively to her needs, should not be a hospital employee and should have no conflicting responsibilities. Support is best begun before a woman is in active labour and the pain is a challenge. For it to work best she must be able to say what she wants – when she wants it. Rather than being on the receiving end of care, she is collaborating with her birth companion and they work closely together.

The suggestions I make in Chapter 5 regarding how a midwife, a birth partner and a doula should give emotional support during childbirth can help a companion fill a vital role for any woman giving birth.

There are many ways to handle pain without drugs, most of which entail discussion and preparation beforehand. For some of these a helper with expert skills is necessary.

CUTANEOUS INJECTION OF STERILE WATER

This medical intervention was first introduced by Dr Michel Odent to treat kidney pain, and subsequently for severe backache in labour at approximately 5 centimetres dilatation of the cervix.[122] It is a technique used by Swedish obstetricians. The pain relief lasts for at least 45 minutes. No side effects have been observed. 'A large trial showed that compared with drugs for pain relief water injections reduced the chance of Caesarean section.'[123,124] The disadvantage is a sharp stinging pain as the water is injected and for up to half a minute after. Entonox can be inhaled during this time. This method of pain relief needs to be discussed with the obstetrician or midwife beforehand, as it is a method that is not usually employed.

TRANSCUTANEOUS ELECTRONIC NERVE STIMULATION (TENS)

A TENS machine consists of four sticky electrode pads that are applied above and below the waist on either side of the spine and a small hand-held unit that lets the woman operate it herself. Between contractions it is set to provide electronic impulses in 'burst mode', with a pulse rate of 70 or more and a pulse width of 100–150. It feels like a beating heart. The idea is that it helps to stimulate the natural endorphins flowing in the blood that reduce the sensation of pain. When a contraction starts, the woman presses a booster button and the unit switches into continuous mode, producing a sensation like pins and needles. This acts as counter-stimulation to the contraction. At the end of the contraction she presses the booster button so that the machine returns to burst mode. An advantage of TENS is that it is a method under the control of the woman. It is most likely to be of help before 6 centimetres dilatation of the cervix.

For details of how to hire a TENS machine see 'Useful addresses' (pp. 169–73).

ACUPUNCTURE, ACUPRESSURE, SHIATSU AND REFLEXOLOGY

Acupuncture may also be an option. This can be done using fine needles in the traditional Chinese way or with electrode stimulation.[125,126,127,128] In China acupuncture is even used in Caesarean sections. It stimulates production of endorphins, the body's natural painkillers.

Acupressure is a variant in which the thumb and fingers are used. Acupuncture points are stimulated in the sacro-lumbar region, just above the buttocks (avoiding the bone), at the side of the pelvis, on the outside lower leg, at either side of the neck, on the back of the hand between the thumb and index finger, and on the soles of the feet to the side and slightly below the fleshy ball under the big toe.

A traditional Japanese method of using touch, gentle pressure and massage, shiatsu can be used by a birth partner who has studied the technique or a shiatsu specialist. It means literally 'finger pressure'. But the practitioner may also use palms, elbows and knees. Like acupuncture, it is based on the concept of the body as an energy system that includes physical, emotional and spiritual elements.[129,130]

Reflexology is an ancient method of relaxing massage and pressure from fingers and thumb on the feet. The theory is that each part of the body is mapped on the feet.[131]

For more details see 'Useful addresses' (pp. 169–73).

Self-hypnosis is very effective for some women. Up to 20 per cent of people can be hypnotised easily, the same proportion are resistant, while the rest respond with varying degrees of ease. You can test yourself to find out if hypnosis could be useful for you. This is the lemon test:

Sit comfortably and ask your partner to read the following script to you:

Close your eyes and take a deep breath. Exhale slowly. Imagine that you see a plump, yellow lemon on a table. Reach down and pick it up. Now hold it up to your nose and breathe in its citrus fragrance. Put it on the table and slice the lemon in half. See the juice drip out onto the table. Lift half the lemon and squeeze it into a glass. Watch the juice drip from the pulp. Raise the glass and take a sip, allowing the tart, citrus juice to wash over your tongue.

Are you salivating? Many people actually pucker and salivate when they focus on the mental image of tasting a lemon. As you might expect, the better you are at responding to the visual image, the more likely you are to respond to hypnotic suggestions.[132]

Though 'hypnos' is the Greek for 'sleep', it is not necessary to enter a state of trance. Self-hypnosis is a form of relaxed concentration that can be used in preparation for birth, though it helps to have a birth partner who understands the techniques. Steven Griffiths, a hypnotherapy practitioner, says, 'For every thought and emotion there is a physical response. Nature can stop labour if a woman is under threat' and he gives the example of Professor Niles Newton's research in mice. They go out of labour if pads soaked with cat urine are put in their cage. 'A build up of lactic acid causes pain, labour is slowed and the blood supply is reduced.' Researchers suggest that:

Hypnosis somehow causes the frontal limbic system of the brain, which regulates body functions, to inhibit pain impulses from the thalamus (the sensory relay centre of the brain) to the cortex (the part of the brain that handles the perception of sensory information). In other words, hypnosis actually alters the way the brain experiences pain.[133]

OTHER WAYS OF HANDLING PAIN

Self-hypnosis can be learned one-to-one from a hypnotherapist in pregnancy or from CDs aimed at overcoming fear associated with birth, learning deep relaxation and rhythmic breathing, building confidence in your body and developing effective pain management techniques. The CDs often come with relaxing birth music, too, to be used when rehearsing the birth. Listening to them during labour stimulates the positive mental images and deep relaxation that have been practised earlier. For more details see 'Useful addresses' (pp. 169–73).

You could make your own audiotape instead. Go inside yourself and draw from any vivid memories of happy personal experiences. Create a store of these to focus on in childbirth.

When a woman has challenged anxiety in these ways and learned the skills of hypnotherapy in pregnancy, she does not necessarily require a hypnotherapist with her during labour. But she does need to negotiate care so that she can use hypnotherapy. It is difficult to use self-hypnosis if she has regular vaginal examinations and blood pressure checks, and instructions about how she should breathe or positions she should adopt. So it helps to have a midwife who is positive about hypnotherapy and can enhance its effects.

TOUCH RELAXATION AND MASSAGE

This is the method of positive body awareness that I developed as a way of working *with* pain instead of fighting it. Fear and anxiety are readily communicated through touch, so it is important that whoever is offering massage is someone the mother trusts and with whom it is easy to relax, ideally a close friend or partner – and it is also important that that person is confident and relaxed. It is best if massage for labour is practised during pregnancy, so that a language of non-verbal communication is created between the two people involved. Massage should be slow, firm, and given with oiled hands moulded to the shape of the body. The message from the hand is always, 'Relax here, now, letting any tension flow out towards the warmth of my touch.' In this way it actively stimulates a woman to relax. She does not simply *receive* massage. It is interactive. She enters into a dialogue with whoever is helping her.

When I first introduced this interactive massage in *The Experience of Childbirth*, I called it 'Touch Relaxation' and it is described fully in *The New Experience of Childbirth*.[134] The aim is to bypass words and use other forms of stimulus. The grammar of this non-verbal language of touch is simple: the woman releases towards the touching hand.

Practising touch relaxation

To practise touch relaxation, you need to contract a muscle, and when you are ready, your birth partner rests a hand over it. As this happens, release the muscle, flowing out *towards* the hand. Some ways to do this are:

- Frown. Your partner rests a hand on your brow. Relax.
- Grit your teeth and clench your jaw. The helper rests a hand on either side of your jaw. Relax.
- Raise your eyebrows. Your helper rests hands on either side of the skull. Relax.
- Press your shoulder blades back as if they were an angel's wings and you can make them touch each other. Your partner rests a hand at the front of each shoulder. Relax.
- Pull in your abdominal wall towards your spine. Your partner rests both hands over the lower curve of your abdomen. Relax.
- Press your upper legs together as if you could hold a sheet of paper between them. Your partner cradles a hand round the outside of each leg. Relax as your legs flop apart.
- Press your legs out, forcing your thighs apart. Your partner rests a hand on the inside of each thigh. Relax.
- Contract the muscles of an arm like a wooden doll, fingers stretched out. Your partner first rests both hands firmly on your shoulder and inner upper arm, then slowly, with one hand still on the shoulder, runs the other hand down the arm on the inside, and you relax completely.
- Contract the muscles of a leg, pointing your toes up towards the ceiling and straightening your leg (but not if it gives you cramp). Your helper places one hand over the inside of your upper leg and the other over the outside, moulding both to the shape of your body. Relax your leg. Then, slowly and deliberately with a long stroke, your partner moves both hands down the leg to the ankle, ending with one hand holding your bare foot firmly round the instep. All residual tension flows out, as if into the cradling hand.

Other exercises that can be done lying on your side are:

- Lift your chin in the air and contract muscles at the back of your neck. Your partner rests a hand in the nape of your neck and you relax.

- Hollow your lower back. Your helper rests both hands either side of the sacro-lumbar spine and you relax.
- Press your buttocks together tightly. Your partner rests a hand over the curve of each buttock and you relax.

Types of massage

These are the types of massage I have found most effective in helping women at different times during childbirth:

- Massage of the sacro-lumbar area is helpful when the birth companion kneads the small of the woman's back, exerting pressure from the heel of the hands. It does not work well if the hands just slip over the flesh. It needs to be deep and firm. This kind of massage helps when a woman has acute back pain.
- Long, stroking movements with both hands down the back from shoulders to buttocks can feel good, too. The helper should avoid massaging over the spine, and keep to either side of it. A continuous, flowing movement is simple if one hand is starting on a shoulder as the upper hand reaches the lower back.
- Massage of the buttocks as if kneading bread dough helps relieve pain as the pressure of the baby's head gets lower.
- Shoulder massage, keeping the hands on the shoulders and using the thumbs for deep massage, is useful if the woman's breathing threatens to run away with her and she is panting fast and furiously.
- Legs often tense up in labour. Facing the woman, the partner massages the inner thighs with elbows raised, from the top of the legs to the knees. This also helps release pelvic floor muscles and is helpful during transition between the first and second stages.
- Foot massage can be done with hands grasping the balls of the feet, applying pressure with the thumbs. Again, this is helpful if contractions threaten to take a woman's breath away. It enables her to keep her breathing rhythmic.
- Abdominal massage should only ever be done very lightly. The woman herself, or her partner, can stroke the area over the dilating cervix with a light touch. It is best done as if gently stroking the baby's head, curving from one side down towards the pubis, and up a little at the other side, one hand following on the other in a continuous stroking movement.

WAYS A WOMAN CAN HANDLE PAIN HERSELF

An important approach to handling pain is to challenge fear. To do that, a woman needs to understand what causes the pain, have accurate information about it, and know what intensifies it. She needs to be 'in touch' with the pain – not running away from it. Then she starts to feel that she is in control, rather than being under attack.

Relaxation

Tensing up to pain is a spontaneous reaction, but one that makes pain worse. Pain is a signal to relax. The simplest way to do this is to breathe out, drop shoulders and let tension flow out of the body from the top of the head, all down the spine, and down the legs and arms, feet and hands. It is probably most effective when combined with massage. The mother should control where she is massaged, and exactly how. She is the conductor. The birth companion who is doing the massage takes the lead from her, like an orchestra responding to the conductor.

Breathing

Breathing is naturally associated with relaxation. Long, slow breaths with the emphasis on the breath out, not the breath in, are most effective, allowing a slight pause between the breath in and the breath out, and the breath out and the breath in. This enables relaxation to get deeper and deeper. The tendency is to suck breath in with pain. If pain continues, we start to hyperventilate and the balance between carbon dioxide and oxygen in the blood is lost. So the woman in labour relaxes a little more with each breath *out* and lets the breath in look after itself. Rhythmic breathing, too, may be best combined with massage.

By the end of pregnancy the uterus is an enormous and extraordinarily strong muscle, the size of a large melon. It is larger than the biceps of a champion boxer. When it contracts it is felt as a tight squeeze. For a woman experiencing this for the first time it seems incredible that anything so powerful can be working inside her body, without her willing it or being able to stop it. Contractions share the elemental energy of ocean tides, wind and fire. This is the power of birth.

Visualisation

The power of imagination can be used positively to focus on images, scenes, sounds and feelings that a woman knows relax her. In labour it helps to visualise muscles working, tissues fanning out and opening, a great flower spreading wide all its petals, the baby's head pressing down, and the body working to actively give birth to this child. Some women 'see' contractions in terms of bands of colour spreading, deepening in intensity. Or they create a combined visual and kinetic image – such as swimming over waves, surfing or skiing down a mountainside – that harmonises with the sensations produced by contractions.

This is completely different from 'doing exercises' and is amazingly effective for any woman who can use her imagination in a creative way.

It is hard to concentrate on images in this way if she is in an unsupported and intrusive environment. She needs her own space in which she can focus on these vivid images. It helps a great deal if she has a birth companion or a midwife in a one-to-one relationship with her who can guard that space.

Vocalisation

Vocalisation comes spontaneously. Some women sing. Others moo. Screaming does not help. Even the sound of your own screaming can be frightening. But a long groan or sigh may dissolve pain. Low sounds help to relieve pain. High-pitched sounds intensify it. Writing about her experience of birth, Lauren Slater says:

> I start to sing.
> I never knew such songs existed in me. I never knew, until labor, the power of sound to contain and expel pain . . . When the next contraction comes I open my mouth and low, drawing the sound up from the deepest part of my stomach, and it helps . . .
> This goes on for I don't know how long. I low my way through labor.[135]

Position change

Pain often stimulates a change in position. Backache or abdominal cramp, for example, often results in spontaneous adjustment of posture to reduce the pain, taking pressure off nerve endings. The same thing occurs in labour. Women seek to be upright, on all fours, or to have back support, for example. They do not have to be told to do this. They know what helps relieve pain, and they resist uncomfortable positions, such as lying flat on their backs.

Movement

Acute pain triggers movement. It may be an attempt to move away from the source of pain, which is what happens when we reach into the oven and touch hot metal by mistake, or it may be flapping, slapping or jigging up and down when we stub a toe, for example. In the same way, birth pain stimulates movement – essentially movement of the pelvis and spine. This includes rocking, circling and tilting the pelvis and curling and uncurling the spine.

Movement can be consciously patterned in response to uterine contractions. Birth then becomes a dance. It may be a solo, a dance in the arms of a birth partner, or one supported by a companion on either side. A traditional birth sculpture from Peru shows a woman kneeling and rocking supported by the body of a woman helper behind her. Co-ordinated movement like this can be practised and then adapted to the needs of the moment when she is in labour.

Water

Lying in a bath or having a shower after strenuous exertion is refreshing and eases aching muscles. Immersion in water at a comfortable temperature acts as a counter-stimulus to pain. Women know that warm water often relieves the uterine cramp and backache of menstrual pain. It can also help with labour pain.

Women who labour in a pool use significantly fewer drugs for pain relief.[136,137,138,139,140] One advantage of labouring in water is that it is easy to move freely if the pool is large enough. Not only does water enable the woman to float but she can turn, change the angle of her pelvis and 'dance' in the water.

Warmth

Just as warm water is relaxing, so are hot compresses, hot-water bottles or the kind of wheat or rice packs that can be heated in the microwave. They can feel good in the small of the back, against the inner thighs, or at the back of the neck.

Any woman who decides that she needs analgesic drugs or an epidural has not failed. In the circumstances she has made a choice that, given the pain she is experiencing, is right at the time. Everything that happens afterwards – interventions that occur despite her hopes – are part of an obstetric chain of events over which she has no control. If she has managed to push her baby out in spite of an epidural, she can feel victorious. If she has managed to deliver vaginally with instruments, she can feel victorious. If she has had a Caesarean section and fallen in love with her baby, she can feel triumphant, too. Breastfeeding in spite of all she has been through is a brilliant achievement.

But suppose she has not managed to do any of these things, looks back on the birth as a chaotic ordeal and feels alienated from her baby? Facing up to – acknowledging – trauma, putting it all into words, is a courageous act in which she sets out on a journey of healing where she is in control – born of her inner strength.

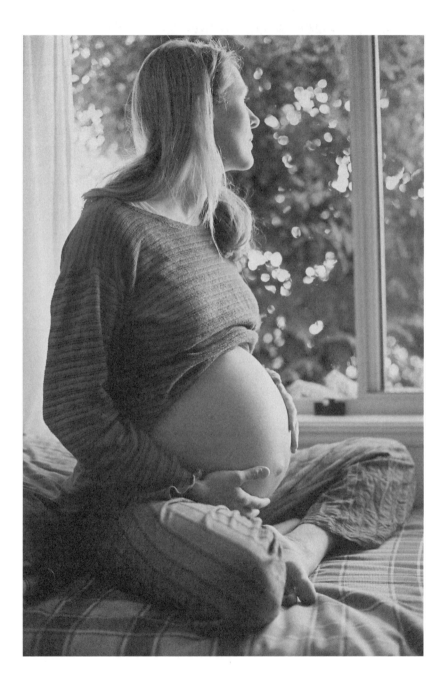

'IF ONLY I HADN'T'

9

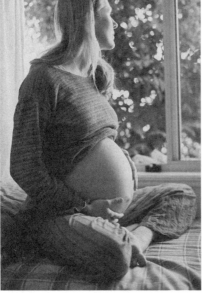

E VERY ONE OF US has been through experiences in life on which we look back and think, 'If only I hadn't . . .' This may be realistic regret. We wouldn't have done it that way with the knowledge we have now. We can learn from it. But sometimes regret mutates into pervasive guilt and stops us moving forward. We are consumed by it. This is how it may be for a woman after a distressing birth experience:

> *I want to have a normal life. I'm hurting my marriage and causing damage to my son but I don't know what to do. It's just a round of failure, feeling guilty, being very defensive.*

*I felt all of the control had been taken off me. I felt powerless
and guilty for wanting a Caesarean.*

*I feel very guilty about the way I view my first birth. My experi-
ence of motherhood this time round is so much calmer and
breastfeeding is going brilliant. I gave up after eight weeks with
my first. I have bonded immediately and I feel bad, because I
love both my daughters the same. I can barely speak the words
that this birth was so much more superior, which I hate myself
for thinking. I feel such a bad mum.*

After a traumatic birth that ends in a forceps or ventouse delivery
or an emergency Caesarean section – and in rare cases in the baby's
death – a woman often blames herself. She feels she was inadequate
or defective. It wouldn't have happened that way if she had been
stronger, more determined, better informed, or more assertive. It was
her failure.

CHOICES

We often make wrong choices or are coerced into submission when
at our most vulnerable in pregnancy and birth. Women sometimes
act out of fear that if they do not follow professional advice or obey
orders the baby will be harmed or they will be punished. This is why
they agree to induction of labour and continuous electronic monitoring and sign the permission form for a Caesarean. They are told
that they should lie in bed, because otherwise the baby's heart cannot
be recorded properly. Most interventions are explained, if they are
explained at all, in terms of the benefit to the baby – never in terms
of the ease of working of institutional protocols, and rarely in terms
of a research project or the training of junior members of staff.

A hospital is like a machine that can only be kept running when
the parts are used regularly. It might grind to a halt if patients did
not have vaginal examinations so that midwives could write up their
records; if women were strolling around the hospital grounds while
the senior obstetrician arrived to examine; if midwives and house
officers did not have systematic practice in interpreting CTG data;
if patients had long, slow labours that resulted in beds being occupied for days; and if midwives were required to leave the hospital
to attend home births when the delivery suite was full.

Because of the shortage of midwives, senior managers are engaged
in a mammoth feat of organisation anyway. So patients cannot be

allowed to step out of line. They can make minor choices, yes, but the hospital culture is dominant and, as we have seen in Chapter 4, sustains itself through institutional norms from which individual practitioners and patients deviate at their peril. It is in the interest of the institution to organise caregivers and patients so that they behave in approximately the same way. Behaviour must be predictable, sanctioned and regulated. Some women have artificial rupture of the membranes, prostaglandins, syntocinon to stimulate the uterus, pethidine and epidurals so that labour is made to conform within standard limits whenever possible. Women are confined to bed so that they are readily available for surveillance. When labour has been speeded up, drugs to deal with pain, often a direct consequence of such interventions, are offered. Uterine activity is stimulated further because painkilling medication has made contractions weaker; then, because there is concern about the baby and the length of time that labour is taking, the decision is made to go for instrumental delivery or, if the theatre is free and a surgeon and anaesthetist available, Caesarean section. That is how most hospitals are run.

Women say, 'It was all my fault. I should never have agreed to it.' Or 'I should have protested.' They often add, 'I didn't know', 'I trusted them.' Sometimes they say that a partner persuaded them to 'trust the professionals'. The question often asked of them, 'Could you ever forgive yourself if something happened to the baby?' implies that they are self-indulgent and reckless.

Bridget had her third baby three years ago and a Caesarean section when she had been in the second stage for an hour and a half.

When she became pregnant again the obstetrician proposed an elective Caesarean, which she refused. It was a highly managed labour – 'They couldn't wait to hook me up' – ending in an emergency Caesarean at which she received a four-inch cut in her bladder. She was given morphine, cannot remember holding the baby, and was in so much pain afterwards that she could neither walk nor breastfeed. People criticised her for being 'dramatic'.

Guilt ranges from self-criticism – 'How *could* I have done that?' to what amounts to self-flagellation. It is often revealed in layers like rock strata. Pam tells me that she is 'very sad and guilty' that she was too tired after a long and difficult second stage to greet her newborn baby. As she talks a deeper anxiety is revealed. She says she was 'sitting on his head' and is now concerned that she may have damaged him, although there is no evidence of it.

When women blame themselves like this they are often affected by the opinions and fears of other people whose anxieties are expressed through a mother they perceive to have put her baby's life at risk.

MATERNAL-FETAL CONFLICT

Doctors are there to save the baby. They are advocates for the fetus. And they often see themselves as the only advocates the fetus has. The theory of maternal-fetal conflict, a battle that takes place between the woman and the fetus for nutrients and very survival, was already popular among doctors in the eighteenth century. Drawings made by Lorenz Heister in 1740 illustrate vigorous babies who put the mother at risk by leaping into all sorts of difficult positions and becoming impacted.

In our contemporary technocratic birth culture we have developed this idea further. Biologists have coined the term 'genetic conflict' to describe difficult pregnancies in which the baby thrives, asserting control over the mother. When a pregnant woman's interests – as she sees them – conflict with those of the fetus, as defined by the obstetrician, there is 'maternal-fetal' conflict. This happens if she does not comply with medical advice. It might be about fetal surgery, a blood transfusion or a Caesarean section. Or it may be because she persists in behaviour that her caregivers consider put the fetus at risk, for example, if she smokes, drinks alcohol, takes drugs, has a bad diet, or won't resign from a job in a hazardous environment.

This medical view of the mother and fetus in a struggle for survival is in direct contrast to a woman's view of pregnancy as an expression of the unity between her and her baby. In traditional cultures pregnancy is perceived as risky, but not because of conflict between the mother and her baby, but of spiritual dangers to both, since they are each in a marginal or transitional state. The logical outcome of the medical paradigm of conflict is that the woman readily becomes both victim of her pregnancy – the fetus a parasite and predator – and also culpable – an irresponsible mother, who attacks and may even destroy the baby. She can be guilty of child abuse while the baby is still *in utero*.

A woman who wants a home birth, one who refuses to be induced or have continuous monitoring, is considered irresponsible and a risk to her baby. Those obstetricians who view the mother and fetus as antagonists believe that they must protect a baby from its mother. Della Pollock in her book on birth narratives writes:

*Death is what medicine overcomes. It is the antagonist van-
quished in a morality play acted out over and over again in birth
stories. Should death occur . . . it must be by some fault of the
mother – some failure to comply with medical exigencies or some
congenital weakness that makes her shamefully immune to
medical help. She must have been rebellious or unsuited from
the outset . . .*[141]

Thus women do not only blame themselves. They are blamed.

WHO'S TO BLAME

Yet accusations go further than that. A woman who has had a
previous Caesarean section and plans a home birth against obstetric
advice, and who is then admitted to hospital because of a complicated labour, may even be at risk of being referred by her caregivers
to social services on the grounds of child abuse. Women try hard
to be grateful. Cherry had a 'crash section' and says:

*I do kind of feel this guilt, I always end up saying 'At least I've
got a healthy baby' and I'm on the mend myself. When I was
in tears because I'd had a Caesarean section with my wee girl
this woman said to me, 'You're so selfish. All you're thinking
about is yourself.' Which wasn't the case. This was someone
who barely knew me.*

She added, 'I'm wondering if things would have been different if I
hadn't had artificial rupture of the membranes.' She told me that
she had made a birth plan but it wasn't discussed because she
accepted diamorphine for the pain 'and I was in such a world of
my own that I forgot to give her my birth plan'.

Women who feel that they do not have the right maternal emotions
and did not bond with the baby at first, or for a long time, express
guilt about this, too: 'I wished that he had never existed and then
feel guilty for thinking such a thing, because none of it was his
fault.' They sometimes use the word 'cheated', too:

*I feel like I've cheated the baby in the first seven weeks of his
life because I haven't been right.*

*I felt guilty as everybody expects for you to have this amazing
mother–daughter bond and I didn't have it! I felt abused! With*

the pain and the horrible post operation recovery that couldn't really let you look after your child properly.

I feel guilty as my best friend has a blind handicapped son who is now three and I am lucky as my son is OK so why am I moaning? I could not breastfeed my son due to lack of milk caused I am told by the birth and subsequent operations. This makes me feel that I have failed him as I could not give birth naturally and could not even feed him. I tried for a month and then had to give up.

I felt cheated that my mum, sister and husband saw my son before me, that I could not feed him and hold him immediately like the other mums on the ward . . . that I could not breastfeed him. I struggled to bond with him and felt incredibly guilty.

After a traumatic birth experience women feel guilty for wanting a home birth, guilty for wanting a Caesarean section, guilty for surrendering control to the medical system, and guilty about resisting medical interventions. Studying their birth stories, there seems no way they can avoid guilt, though when they have a chance to talk about how they feel, many come to terms with it and can move on.

Not every woman who has had an emergency Caesarean section is tortured by guilt, however. One who wrote to me reflected that 'At the time, it seemed to be the safest option' and is grateful to her obstetrician. Told that her baby was breech at 38 weeks, and pregnant with her fifth child, she said that she 'knew immediately that this would mean my first Caesarean section. I cried from shock, from fear and anxiety'. An ultrasound estimated the baby's weight at over 11 pounds, but also revealed that it had turned. After discussion with the obstetrician she decided to go ahead with the Caesarean, partly because she was told that the alternative was to stay in hospital until the birth, and there were the other children to look after.

During surgery the obstetrician cut a vein by mistake and she haemorrhaged. He made another incision to get the baby out quickly, but for some reason this failed. So he did a vertical incision 'blind, due to the large volume of blood I was losing.' The result was a '12cm laceration across the baby's lower back' who had an Apgar score of 5 and later 7 and needed to be on a respirator. He weighed 9 pounds 5 ounces. The mother writes:

'I don't blame anyone . . . It was easy to forgive the obstetrician who seemed genuinely upset and worried . . . and I still hold to

*that.' She felt 'devastated', 'helpless', 'shocked', but says those
words are inadequate. The baby had surgery to repair the wound
five hours later and was baptised before being anaesthetised. 'The
obstetrician came to see me several times that first day. Each
time he updated me. He didn't disappear and let others cover
for him. He was diligent in his care. The worry and devastation
that he was feeling was very evident, and in a strange way it
helped me to cope better.' The baby's wound became infected
and broke down on the third day. 'It had to be packed twice a
day as it was gaping.' At times she was 'frightened' not only for
but of the baby. He was fast losing weight. Then her wound
became infected, so both she and the baby were on antibiotics.
They were discharged two weeks after the birth. The baby's
wound took six weeks to heal. She goes on to say 'Quite a few
people have asked me if I regret having a c-section. With some
thought I have to say no. There are no guarantees in life and at
the time, it seemed to be the safest option.' But she does wonder
if it was necessary. 'I was after all only 38 weeks ... Given a
week or two or three could Nathaniel have turned?' She has been
told by two obstetricians that she must never get pregnant again.
But she ends, 'I am grateful to my doctor for his support, to my
husband, my wonderful friends and family and to God in whom
I will always have unwavering faith.'*[142]

111

The concept of risk is difficult. Any suggestion of risk to the baby
sounds alarm bells in women who want birth to be risk-free. A
woman often feels that if she is a 'good patient', she reduces or
eliminates risk. One told me that she did not want to 'go against
expert medical opinion'. Yet experts may differ. In her case, an obstetrician who had performed a Caesarean with her previous birth
advised her to opt for elective Caesarean section because she had
'a narrow synthesis pubis'. She commented, 'That does put your
confidence into a bit of a crisis.' A second obstetrician said that
the first obstetrician was 'perhaps erring on the side of caution'. She
was afraid of courting disaster and said, 'I don't want to come across
as a defensive, aggressive, battling mother who is obstreperous about
these things.'

Other women are simply glad that obstetric help was available
and are unreflective about why a Caesarean was done. They accept
the medical explanation that it was necessary for the baby's sake.
In fact, sometimes the narrative they construct presents a Caesarean
as the best possible way of birth, superior to other birth experiences.

A woman who had an instrumental delivery for fetal distress resulting in perineal injury (though the baby turned out to have an Apgar score of 9 at birth, so she was sure that it was not necessary for the baby's sake) said, 'I have been hurt by women who have had Caesareans proudly saying that at least their vaginas are still in "perfect nick" or "I am so glad I asked for a Caesarean and didn't have to go through that. I am sure my husband is happy too – we had sex after six weeks."'

One way of seeking to control and devise meaning and significance in life-threatening events is to tell the story. We frame the event in narrative that explains what occurs and describes and justifies our role in it. In the past, myth and fable provided a model for this. Cinderella and Snow White in fairy tales, and Persephone, Ephigenia, Electra and other heroines of Greek legend serve as symbols of women at their most vulnerable. Metaphor enables an individual to have a place in the drama.

Today these metaphors can be drawn from television. A woman may explain and justify the events of birth in the context of a TV soap opera. When they become part of that narrative they understand their role in it, communicate their experiences to others more easily. They are part of a story that has powerful shared meaning; the listener has seen the programmes too. A soap opera can contribute to creating our reality and shaping our views of it. In presenting the metaphor the storyteller is not isolated and in distress, struggling to communicate what happened to her in a unique and extraordinary way. She takes control of the story and gives it the ready-made meaning that she wants the listener to accept.

In a letter to the 'alternative' Canadian magazine *Birthing*, Leah described how her labour was induced because she had a skin condition – PUPPS (pruritic urticarial papules and plaques of pregnancy, an itchy rash on the body that disappears after delivery of the placenta, and does not affect the baby). She says:

It looked like I had the worst case of chickenpox that anybody had ever seen and I couldn't stop scratching! [During labour] the nurse was checking the fetal monitoring strip and looked concerned. Before I knew it two more nurses were in the room, looking at the strip and conferring amongst themselves. At this point I was informed that my baby's heart rate was dropping dangerously low with each contraction. My doctor was called in. He advised me that the drop in heart rate was possibly due to having my membranes ruptured too soon, and that they would be attempting to 'refill' the amniotic sac with saline in hopes that the baby would be cushioned and less stressed. [It didn't work.] The doctor ran to the phone . . . I felt like I was in a movie, when he said, 'Prep the OR – stat!' then over the large intercom, 'Code blue, room 232, code blue,' was ringing through the hallways. None of us had any idea what was going on. It was just like a scene from ER. Eight doctors and nurses came out of the wood-work into my room. Cords were flying everywhere, an oxygen mask was put on my face and I was given medication to stop the contractions. My doctor then told me that my baby had a 'pro-lapsed cord'. I was in the operating theatre in a matter of minutes, the epidural was in place extremely quickly . . . I have never per-sonally witnessed doctors working so quickly and efficiently. Despite her traumatic entrance into this world, she is now a per-fectly healthy and happy 6-year-old. It is true that not a lot of women want to brag about their surgical births, but I certainly like to brag about mine. I am eternally grateful to those nurses who caught the drop in the heart rate, and more so to the doctor who I can say saved my child's life. [143]

HOW TO LISTEN

Some counsellors and therapists seek to explain guilt after a trau-matic birth as being due to early childhood trauma. Maybe. It is difficult to produce evidence. There must be very few people who have not experienced childhood trauma. If a woman does not choose the route of psychoanalysis, hypnosis, re-birthing and dream analysis, it is better to stick with the here and now.

Explaining suffering in terms of childhood trauma and errors in parenting can be extremely irritating, too. Hannah said a counsellor told her that:

I wouldn't have interpreted the events of my daughter's birth in the way I have, and they wouldn't have been traumatic, unless I have unresolved past traumatic experiences. My parents' divorce has caused my sense of existential loneliness, for example (it couldn't be that I felt like a passive witness to my own child's birth, completely absent actually, who was born into the world alone). How silly of me to even consider this as a possibility. Or course it must be my parents' divorce. This is outrageous to me. My baby was in a life and death situation. I watched her gasping for air, being resuscitated, her eyes rolling back in her

head, machines which were sustaining her life shutting down,
equipment and medicines not being available for her, the two
babies that shared her room dying in front of my eyes. I wanted
to die if she died. She is almost three and I am frozen in that
state of terror from her birth. Isn't this experience traumatic
enough in itself? I am left feeling like some horrible, ugly, selfish
person for feeling this way. I feel so angry. My anger, selfish-
ness, immaturity, naivety . . . I know it isn't the worst thing that
anyone has experienced in the world, but don't I count for
anything? The words that I have heard from people just ring in
my ears, 'She's alive isn't she? There is nothing wrong with her
now? Be responsible for your child.' This last set of counselling
appointments is just leaving me feeling like there is no one in
the world who can help me.'

Hannah needed me to address the issues that faced her now, not
incidents in her past, even if they have become an important part
of her. She told me, 'I miss *me.*' She didn't want to discover her
inner child. She needed to find herself again as an adult.

As you listen to a woman who bitterly regrets choices she made
or things that were done to her that she felt helpless to resist, you
may sometimes get a niggling question in your own mind, 'Yes,
why didn't you?' That way lies criticism and judgement. Suggestions
about what she could and should have done if things were different
– if she had been you and not her – are worse than useless.

Head-on confrontation with guilt is pointless. I have learned that
when I say 'You don't have to feel guilty' or 'It's not your fault'
a woman will protest, 'I know, but I do!' and think of reasons
why she should feel guilty, whatever I say. It is better to acknowledge the guilt that we *all* feel about losing control, letting ourselves
be bullied, trusting someone whom we should not have trusted,
guilt for our ignorance in a situation where we needed to *know*,
for being unable to stand up for ourselves about what we believe,
or making a choice that later proved to be disastrous. This is the
gist of how the recorded conversation went with one woman who
phoned me in distress, and gave her consent to quote the discussion
between us:

EVE   *I just found the whole thing absolutely petrifying.*
SHEILA *Oh, I can imagine.*
EVE   *When I came round from the anaesthetic I can remember*
         I was screaming at that point and I was terrified that either

I was dead or the baby was dead . . . I wrote to the hospital
and I asked them what happened, you know. Was it something
with the anaesthetic, was it that I wasn't – somehow I wasn't
– brave enough to cope with a Caesarean, and they sort of
said 'Well it could be either'.

SHEILA   *Oh really!*

EVE   *And so I've still sort of harboured the feeling that, you know,*
that maybe it was kind of all my fault.

SHEILA   *Yes.*

EVE   *If I'd allowed them to break my waters earlier, maybe the*
baby's head would've come down. If I'd had a higher pain
threshold or a greater mental tolerance.

SHEILA   *We always do blame ourselves, don't we?*

Another mother, Fiona, was having flashbacks and panic attacks.
She 'nearly passed out' at the doctor's when her baby was being
given an injection:

FIONA   *I just freaked out.*

SHEILA   *It's very understandable. It doesn't sound to me abnormal*
at all. It sounds to me a rather normal reaction. I think I
might've reacted in much the same way.

FIONA   *That's nice to hear. Because I just felt I was just being a bit*
melodramatic about the whole thing.

SHEILA   *No. I don't see that at all.*

FIONA   *I'm really lucky because I did have a rupture and my son was*
very lucky to be alive. I have been told that I should be
grateful for small mercies.

SHEILA   *I'm sure people who tell you that haven't been through*
anything like that.

FIONA   *And I'm just so bloody angry about it.*

SHEILA   *Yes, and control was taken from you completely. You take a*
baby for an injection and other people take over.

FIONA   *That's it exactly. I didn't think of that.*

SHEILA   *It's like re-enacting the situation but on a minor scale.*

FIONA   *Here you are. Here's the sacrificial altar. Here's my*
son.

SHEILA   *That's right.*

FIONA   *No I didn't think of it like that. I just thought I was being*
hysterical.

SHEILA   *It's a pity you blame yourself.*

FIONA   *I wish I'd been stronger.*

115

SHEILA	*Yes, it's very, very easy looking back on situations to think 'I wish I'd been stronger. I wish I'd done that.' The point is, those things happened and you did whatever you could under the circumstances to the best of your ability.*
FIONA	*You're right. And we always could've done more, I suppose.*
SHEILA	*Yes, yes, and none of us are perfect, and we all have ideals of behaviour, don't we? And some of us drive ourselves a bit about it and demand an awful lot of ourselves.*
FIONA	*Thank you for saying that. Nobody <u>else</u> has said that. Nobody else is involved.*

Each of us has had to act, to make decisions to submit to someone else's decisions, at points in our lives where we have had limited information. We may have known what it is like to be sucked into a medical system in which we were as insignificant as specks of dust. As mothers we blame ourselves for everything that happens to our children. We are responsible. We may suspect that even a child who seems perfect has been scarred by a difficult birth or our failure to bond in the first hours, days – or months.

Cathy has been having panic attacks since the birth of her second child. She had a retained placenta and the doctor ruptured her uterus with a scalpel in an attempt to remove it:

CATHY	*I didn't see her for three days after that. I'd already had a baby a couple of years before that and I missed what I thought was the crucial time for my bonding with it.*
SHEILA	*Yes, of course.*
CATHY	*For six years now I've waited to come out of this dark tunnel. [She starts to sob.] I'm waiting to be back to the person I used to be. I don't feel I've bonded with Susie. Like I should have.*
SHEILA	*I'm sorry.*
CATHY	*And I didn't know whether it was because she was a demanding baby. She wasn't particularly a demanding baby, but as a toddler she became very wilful. But I never took time to play with her or do things with her that I could with my other daughter. I just went through the motions. And I still feel that I just go through the motions. I don't actually <u>mother</u> my children like I feel I should. And I am very alone. And very <u>frightened</u>. [She weeps uncontrollably. Sheila waits. Then Cathy continues.] I was going to go to the doctor this week just to get me something to get me through this Christmas because I don't want this Christmas to happen. I didn't think*

>   *I could cope with it . . . I don't have any relations with my*
>   *husband any more. And it's <u>me</u>. It's not him. It's <u>me</u>.*
>   *And I detach myself from him <u>and</u> the children.*
> SHEILA   *Well, you feel it's the only way to protect yourself I suppose.*
> CATHY   *I have to stay back.*

Cathy talks about her own childhood, how her mother also had a traumatic birth, and everyone in the family has 'sorted things out on their own'. She continues:

> CATHY   *I'm waiting for the day they turn around and blame me.*
>   *Because it will happen if I don't change now.*
> SHEILA   *Yes, but remember all children blame their parents for things*
>   *that go wrong.*
> CATHY   *Do they?*
> SHEILA   *I think so. Yes, I think so. We can't be <u>perfect</u> mothers. You*
>   *sound a pretty <u>good</u> mother.*
> CATHY   *Well, I don't feel I am . . . and I find those feelings really hard*
>   *to deal with.*
> SHEILA   *Yes, of course.*
> CATHY   *The guilt is just <u>tremendous</u>. And if I don't do something now,*
>   *it will just get worse and worse and worse.*
> SHEILA   *The very fact that you want to reach out and do something*
>   *about it is the very beginning of healing. I'm sure of that.*
>   *And it has to come from you, not somebody <u>telling</u> you that*
>   *you ought to. You know? [Sheila suggests that she seek*
>   *counselling.] A counsellor should be a woman who is a*
>   *mother herself ideally. You don't want a man. You don't want*
>   *somebody who goes back over your early childhood . . .*
> CATHY   *No I don't.*
> SHEILA   *. . . as if that accounts for it, do you?*
> CATHY   *Definitely not.*
> SHEILA   *Somebody who deals with the <u>here</u> and <u>now</u>. And who really*
>   *<u>validates</u> what you feel about this birth – and what went*
>   *wrong. You need to be believed. That's the very beginning of*
>   *it, and work from there, I think.*

Cathy goes on to talk about her family:

> CATHY   *I know my mum herself had a difficult birth with my brother.*
>   *And I know she had quite a traumatic time. She hadn't told me*
>   *about it.*

SHEILA	*How did she handle it, do you know?*
CATHY	*The same way as all my family handle everything. We just live with it.*
SHEILA	*I wonder if it would be a good idea for you to have a talk with her, when you can be quiet together over the washing up or something like that. It may be that <u>she</u> needs to talk, too. And it could be that it's a help to <u>you</u>.*
CATHY	*Yes. Yes, I will. I often feel my Mum's got such a lot of her own things to deal with. Everybody has their own problems and they don't need mine.*
SHEILA	*It's not so much offloading, I think, as <u>sharing</u>.*

FEELINGS OF GUILT

Sometimes talking with a mother or a partner's mother about how it feels to give birth provides a new bridge of understanding between women. The older woman may have bottled up inside her strong feelings that remain with her after many years, and feel inhibited from or ashamed about voicing them. It can be a great relief when at last she can be honest about them. She may not have been able to put into words what the experience of birth was – even to herself. Now the two women can communicate and explore together one of the most intense events in their lives.

Some women find a way through guilt by arguing with themselves (with varying success) that obstetric intervention was nothing to do with them and that they could not have affected the outcome one way or the other. A woman who had an emergency Caesarean section following induction of labour and an epidural, leading to deep transverse arrest, thought it was inevitable and nothing to do with the way the labour was managed. It was the baby who had caused the problems.

Guilt is often associated with anger towards a partner whom the woman perceives as also having failed: 'I'm angry because he didn't stand up for me'; 'He failed to notice what I needed more than anything – that I needed his love and respect and encouragement through words. Why didn't he say anything? My husband, my birth partner, failed me.' Sometimes it is a woman birth companion or a midwife who became a trusted friend in pregnancy whom she feels let her down.

We need to listen and accept this without judgement. But discussion may develop so that you can ask, 'How do you think he/she feels about it?' It may emerge that this person feels guilty, too, but is trying to cope with it in a different way. 'What happens when you talk together about it?'

When a woman has already been through a birth ordeal, followed by self-criticism, she is likely to be better prepared with the next pregnancy. Because she knows how she can be coerced into acquiescence she is determined to do things differently. She goes to another hospital or has a home or birth centre birth. She chooses other caregivers. She is coming to terms with her guilt about the last birth by planning ahead for the next one, and this action can itself contribute to healing. She may be very unsure of the outcome and anxious about it. But she is doing something to help herself, and should be praised for this.

She is likely to find that other people cannot understand her anxiety or her need to plan meticulously. Those who are giving her antenatal care may be critical of her concern to plan carefully. Indeed, they may imply she is over-anxious and emotionally unstable. The Caesarean she had was necessary. She should be grateful that her baby was saved. When Louise wrote a complaint to the hospital, a letter came saying that it was all her own fault and that she was traumatised after birth because of her excessively high expectations. She had been unrealistic and, it implied, self-centred and concerned only with her own emotions – not the baby's safety and the dismissive reactions of the professionals (from her experience) that make it worse. These women are caught up in a vortex of shame and self-blame.

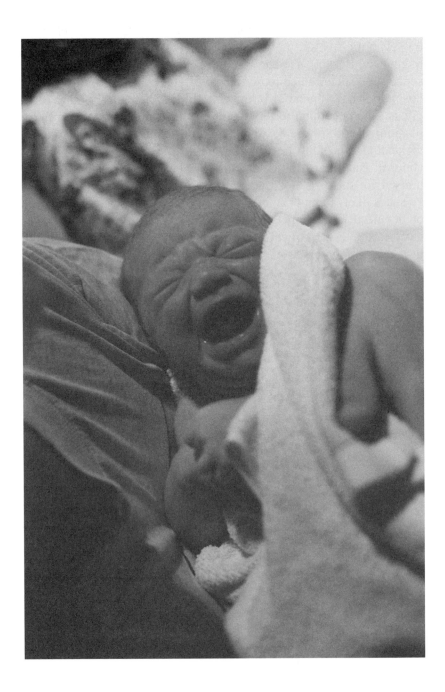

THE BABY

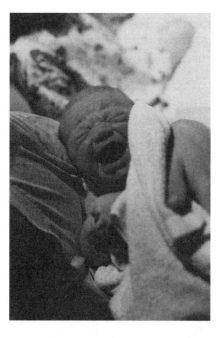

10

WOMEN WHO TALK TO ME about a traumatic birth usually do not focus on the baby. They feel the need to talk about themselves. When I ask about the baby, they say something like, 'The baby's fine – but what about *me*?' or 'It's me I'm worried about.' This seems often to be the one opportunity to focus on their needs instead of acting the part of the good mother and devoting all their attention to the baby.

It is surprising, given the sheer hard work of mothering, that women may refer to the baby only in passing or not at all. In fact, they are more likely to talk about the pregnancy and contrast its ease, and how positive they felt during that time, with the dreadful birth experience. Some, however, have had a difficult pregnancy, and this is often associated with multiple scans, following an anomaly scan that suggested that something was wrong with the baby. They turned up to have the scan believing that this was a celebratory opportunity to 'see the baby' and take an ultrasound photograph or video home with them, only to discover that there was professional concern about thickening at the back of the baby's neck, a cyst in the kidneys or symptoms of other kinds of disability. This anxiety then follows them through pregnancy, the birth and often afterwards, even when the baby appears to be normal.

Some are apologetic about the focus on their own needs: 'Don't think I don't love him. He's a super little boy.' Or 'I love her to bits!' Others, aware of their shift of focus from the baby, say they feel guilty about it and are concerned that they will be accused of being selfish.

TRYING TO BE A GOOD MOTHER

Sometimes it is the baby, and the developing relationship with him, that helps a woman through the experience of post-traumatic stress. It makes it all worthwhile. It is part of the healing.

Yet some women who are traumatised by birth find it very hard to relate to their babies. They feel they are 'not really' a mother and cannot behave like one. They *act* the part and see themselves as robots unable to respond in an emotionally positive and sponta-neous way. A woman sometimes blames the baby for her distressing birth experience:

> He wasn't worth it. I'm told I should be grateful. But I can't help feeling if it weren't for it I wouldn't have had to go through all that. It makes me feel very guilty. Because, of course, it wasn't his fault.

She guards herself against the intensity of her emotions by trying not to feel anything. She simply goes through the motions of mother-ing, feeding, changing nappies, holding, settling down, dressing and undressing, as if the baby did not really belong to her. She may say that she feels as if it has been borrowed. She has no special bond with it: 'I can't stop thinking about the birth. The baby's fine. But I don't feel as bonded with him as I should. Every time I look at him I remember. I feel I really hate him.' Another told me, 'They say, "Be grateful you've got a beautiful baby." But – I've never said this to anyone before – I'd rather my baby had died than I'd have to go through that.'

After a forceps delivery and the birth of a baby with 'a swollen eye and busted lip – I cannot tell you how hideous he looked', the mother could not bring herself to hold him. She said, 'I was completely in shock . . . I even called social services to get them to take my son away.' Now that he is three years old she wants to have another baby, 'But ideally I'd like it to arrive by Parcelforce. It's taken every urge out of me to ever be pregnant again. It scares me.'

A woman who had an emergency Caesarean section under general anaesthetic tells me that she was actually awake, but could not speak or tell the anaesthetist that she could feel the surgeon cutting. She says, 'I can describe the conversation they were having' and continues, 'It is difficult for me to accept the baby as my own. It was if she had been plucked from a tree.'

Another woman who also had a Caesarean, following artificial stimulation of her uterus with a syntocinon drip, wanted very much to breastfeed, but was unsuccessful: 'I feel so robbed . . . but she was sucking and not getting anything, so they cup fed her. Everything was taken out of my hands. I don't feel like she belongs to me.' When a baby has been removed to the nursery for an extended time it can be especially hard. A woman who had what she says was a 'horrendous' Caesarean section told me:

> I'm frightened my brain is going to go. My little boy was taken away. I had problems getting access to him. They gave him to his Dad and took him to Special Care. I wasn't allowed to see him for 12 hours. I'm just going through the motions of being a mother. I look after him. Don't think I'm a bad mother! But I don't get any joy out of it.

In many hospitals babies are removed for observation as a matter of protocol after a Caesarean section. But they may also be taken when a vaginal birth has been complicated. A woman who was induced with prostaglandin pessaries because she was four days past her due date and her blood pressure was slightly raised had a one-and-a-half-hour labour:

> It went hell for leather. My boyfriend pushed the emergency button. Doctors and nurses were running round the room. The midwife got panicky. She was shaking. They were shouting at

her to 'Turn it! Turn it!' I wanted to hold the baby, but they wrapped it up and took it away.

Though her baby is now grown up, this is how Kirsty remembers her daughter's birth:

After heaving and poking about by a variety of gown clad figures, it was over, a baby was pulled out 'from the wreckage', as it were . . . I dimly saw a bundle passed from one gowned figure to another, who was already doing something to the baby as he held her towards me to see, and in the next instant he was putting her in an incubator by the bed. David had returned in time to see the baby emerging, and was at my side watching with me as the paediatrician fiddled with the bundle in the trolley. 'What is it?' I had asked. It was as if we'd all forgotten about that. It didn't seem in the least bit important to know the baby's sex. All that mattered for me was that at last the ordeal was over and the baby seemed to be alive. Someone looked and announced, 'A girl!' I dimly felt enough interest to smile at David.

The next day, they went to see the baby:

Through the glass could be seen a room full of incubators, all containing tiny naked babies with wires running from them. David took me as close as possible to the one he said was ours, and I peered through the glass, trying to take in the knowledge that this baby was mine, this was what had come out of my body the previous day. It was like viewing something in the shop window. None of it seemed real. It still felt as if it were all a dream. How could we know this was our baby? . . . Later that day I went down to see Rosie again through the glass window. Still she lay motionless, sleeping peacefully, her skin pink, unblemished, perfect apart from the raw red bruise on her face. But I felt detached from her – as if I was looking at a doll in a shop window.

Felicity prepared herself for a natural birth, but had forceps, catheters, an epidural and an episiotomy. She says she felt 'envious and cheated':

I didn't feel a thing. My experience left me disconnected from her. During pregnancy I felt as if I knew every inch of her. When she was born I felt sore and angry. I did not feel as if I could identify with her.

The alienation a woman may feel for her newborn is contrasted with the intimacy she experienced in pregnancy. Only when her baby gazes straight into her eyes is the bond re-established, but even then, the baby's needs can seem too much for her to respond to:

> *When I woke the next day I was still weak and sore. I turned over in bed to see a tiny baby staring straight at me. She was wide-eyed, and looking at me with such high expectations. I was suddenly very afraid of the responsibility before me.*

Disruption of the early relationship between mother and baby can have lasting effects. For some of these mothers the baby remained 'it' through the first weeks of life.

Bonding with an unborn baby in the next pregnancy may be difficult, too. A pregnant woman describes this:

> *I'm trying not to think about it, not to let my mind dwell on how awful it was. But now this baby's started moving and I think, 'I don't want you.' It is as if I have been taken over again, and it's all happening again. I can't bear to feel the movements.*

However, when a woman is given confident emotional support, distress at failing to bond gradually gives way to joy in the baby, and she realises that, after all, she has fallen in love.

BONDING

A woman who had described to me how after a traumatic birth she felt on autopilot, could not really mother her baby and was unable to breastfeed wrote enthusiastically when he was seven months old to tell me how wonderful he was and how much she was enjoying him. There was no question of her lacking maternal feelings. She had had the support of family and friends, who assured her, even when she most doubted it, that she was a good mother. She is still having nightmares but fewer of them, 'and I no longer feel guilty that I didn't love him instantly'.

Some women who experience physical disability after childbirth are unable to handle the baby easily – to change nappies, dress and undress and bathe it, for example, and this, too, causes grief. A woman who had back pain and was told by her GP to 'take aspirin and it'll go after a while', said that after a year she was still in agony. 'It goes on and on . . . I still can't lift her. When my mother comes she holds her and rocks her and I feel so envious that she can do things for my baby that I can't do.'

In *Love Works Like This* Lauren Slater tells the story of her induced labour that ends in a Caesarean. She does not meet her baby until the next day, when she is brought to her 'swaddled in several vintage looking cloth blankets, which I love, and which would make for some very snazzy hand towels in my vintage bathroom back at home' with a blue strip 'the exact periwinkle of my shower curtain'. All she can think of is that she would like some of those blankets:

> *'Are we allowed to take the receiving blankets home with us?'*
> *I ask the nurse again.*
> *She frowns, shrugs, 'Not really', she says, 'Is this your first?'*
> *'First and last', I say.*
> *'It takes some time', she says.*[144]

Twenty days after the birth she writes:

> *I am a mother, but I don't look like a mother. I don't feel like a mother. Over and over during the day, or at night when I watch her sleep, I whisper, "I am a mother, mother, mother," as I did when I was pregnant, and I've grown accustomed to the word, but it stays at a distance from me. I thought I would be smashed flat, or heaved high, mythically altered for this, the most mythic of roles but, shock of all shock, here I am, still me. And the baby? I have come to like her a little bit. That's it. A little bit.*[145]

By the time her baby is four months old Lauren feels like a mother and is falling in love with her baby. *Acting* like a mother, doing all the things that mothers do, she is transformed into a mother.

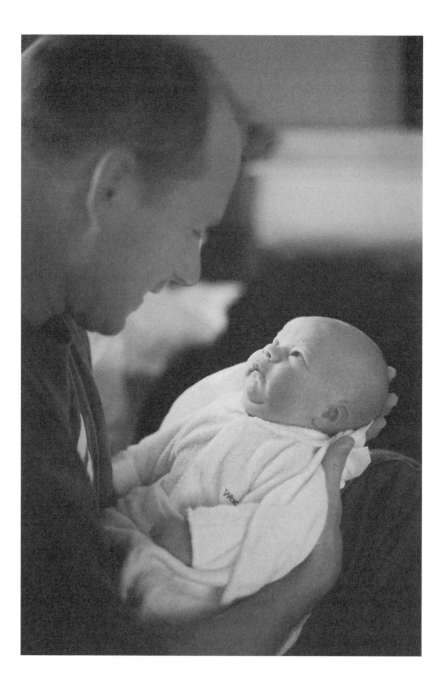

THE PARTNER

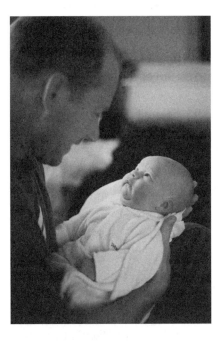

11

'She's had something go wrong with an operation so they say. Some, you know, some internal trouble . . . woman's trouble.'

'The womb, you mean, sir?'

'I don't know do I, Lewis? I didn't ask. I'm not even quite sure where the womb is. And, come to think of it, I don't even like the word.'[146]

M EN MAY BE IGNORANT about 'women's bits', anxious about their potentially leaking effluents and want to leave all that to the professionals. Not only do they know little, but they don't *want* to know.

Those who have had no education for birth may be both embarrassed and frightened by the carnality of birth. Even men who have attended classes often think that they can manage birth – keep it gentle and painless with the right encouraging words and massage in appropriate places – and are shocked when they do not succeed. Men who are confident that they can offer a strong shoulder to lean on are shattered by an experience that is completely out of their control. They feel helpless, sidelined and disempowered.

The experience of birth often has strong impact on a man and woman's perception of themselves, and of each other. When it is positive they are astonished, delighted, fulfilled, feel amazingly clever – and share this euphoria. They are closer together and more in love than ever. It is a peak experience in their relationship.

When a birth has been traumatic this does not happen. It leaves them both shocked, and it can alienate them from each other as they try to deal with the stress, often in different ways. A relationship may break up under the strain.

None of the women who have phoned me for help have been in lesbian relationships. They have all looked to a male partner for support, and many were disappointed: he did not help, could not be relied on, sided with the doctors, succumbed to his own emotions, felt sorry for himself, dismissed her feelings, sloped away when he was most needed, or was a 'voyeur' of a birth, which left her feeling violated. From his point of view, she was irrational, weak and dependent, or changed her mind and didn't stick to the decisions they had made together. She is going on and on about the birth and he can't take any more. As one woman put it, 'My partner says, "The birth is over. Forget it!"'

Each blames the other. This may continue long after the baby is born. Morbidity following birth contributes to the stress, and the combination of having to deal with a woman's physical disability and her distress may cause the relationship to crack under the strain: 'I am trying to forget. But I can't. I don't want to keep raking up the unpleasant. I have often been the worse for drink when my husband gets home from work. He says I'm hysterical.'

Women often comment on their partners' 'patience' and 'understanding' but say it is being stretched to the limit: 'Jack's been ever so patient but I don't think he can stand much more. It's affecting our relationship.'

One woman told me how her first marriage broke up because she was

> so distressed about the terrible experience and we were both
> under such terrific strain ... the two years after the baby was
> born were really dreadful. I couldn't bear him to touch me so
> we split up. She is eight now and I was remarried last spring.
> He wants a baby. I don't know what to do. Perhaps if I could
> have a Caesarean section.

Another woman whose relationship with the father of her baby was also shattered but now has a new partner told me, 'I feel much better now. It's just sad that I will never be able to have another baby. You see, Martin wants children, but I couldn't face going through that again.'

Deanna's baby is a year old now. She told me:

DEANNA *The past year has just been hell. I've just been a mess. It's really affected my relationship with my partner. We've just broken up yesterday.*

SHEILA *Oh, I'm dreadfully sorry. Do you think it's going to be a long-term break-up?*

DEANNA *I don't know. He says that I've become very, very needy.*

SHEILA *Needy?*

DEANNA *Yes. I used to be very independent. I've been very ill. I couldn't look after the baby for the first three months.*

SHEILA *Oh, how dreadful!*

DEANNA *It was horrible. [She tells me her left foot was paralysed for six months.] I've been thinking about having another baby and I'm absolutely terrified it's going to happen again. [She weeps.] I've become very reliant on my partner, which I never was before.*

SHEILA *It's too much for your partner.*

DEANNA *Yes. It's too much for him.*

Sometimes a partner colludes with the professionals who are managing the birth, and a rift occurs in the couple's relationship. A woman whose baby is eight months old says:

I was devastated by the whole thing. I still feel bitter and angry. I can't walk easily. I can't go outside the house. But the worst thing is the effect it has had on my husband. He is traumatised. When they did the delivery they made him help them hold me down. It was brutal. He was shattered by the experience.

Another rang Birth Crisis describing a labour that took place 15 years ago. She had been using Entonox in the second stage, but the midwife took it from her – perhaps so that she would be more alert as she gave birth. Earlier the midwife had told her that she was off duty at 6.30 p.m. There was only a quarter of an hour to go. So she believes that the gas and oxygen was removed so that the midwife could get away. She blames her partner, who is a doctor, for allowing that to happen, and says, 'I've never forgiven him for letting her do it.' She felt emotionally deserted – and this destroyed her trust in him. She did not have another child. 'The fear of pregnancy is affecting my marriage. I get the idea in my head that I'm going to get pregnant. It is such a terrible fear that he might have sneaked up on me in the night.' She has never discussed this with anyone and contacted me because she read an article I had written. 'I thought I was the only person in the world who had this problem. I thought I was alone with it.'

After all these years she is reaching out for help. The horror of a delivery can have a profound effect on the relationship between a couple. A woman had a ventouse delivery that required 36 stitches. Her mother-in-law rang me because she was concerned about her son's distress. The delivery was incredibly painful and the woman's partner hit the doctor and had to be restrained. He blames the baby for the trauma and is determined to have a vasectomy. 'He is so, so, hurt by it all. He just seems to have collapsed.' And she stresses that 'both of them just cry'.

A woman explained to me that she was 'caught between two cultures'. She was herself born in a commune, one of nine children, all of whom had different fathers. She married a doctor, and asked her mother to help with her planned home birth. 'She was great' but her partner was 'driven to distraction' by witnessing her in pain and kept offering pethidine. Because the labour was long, the midwife persuaded her to go into hospital, where she had an epidural and a ventouse delivery. The first attempt failed. With the second attempt she pushed so hard that the baby 'came flying out' and she tore badly. The midwife who sutured her was muttering under her breath, 'Oh, my God, what a mess!' The doctor husband 'went psychotic'. He fled to his parents to be looked after by them and she was left 'alone and frightened'.

SEX

Sex is often difficult for a long time after a distressing birth. This may be because of physical problems – too tight, too loose, too tender, unable to experience orgasm or just total lack of synchronisation – but also because the woman is seething with anger, feels dreadfully let down and cheated, or has low self-esteem and can't enjoy herself through her body any more. She may explain her revulsion from sex in terms of physical changes, and may be right. Yet there is often a strong emotional element, too.

One of the things a woman who is distressed after a vaginal birth often describes is having an episiotomy, being stitched and the after-effects of this. If I ask, 'And sex?', she exclaims, 'There isn't any.'

> *My baby is seven and a half months old now. I have always enjoyed sex, but now each time we make love there is a shooting pain and I have a vision of the doctor who stitched me up. It's horrifying! My doctor shrugs her shoulders and says, 'Oh well, it usually takes a year.' No one gave me any idea of this.*

Jo rang me in distress when her child was three years old. She said the labour was 'fine' until the second stage when 'the midwives were shouting, "Push this baby out or they'll come and cut you!" and verbally abused me. I felt totally threatened – this vision of a man in a white coat with a carving knife.' She had an episiotomy, followed by two failed attempts at ventouse delivery, and then forceps. She feels mutilated and has had long-term perineal problems. She wants another baby, but can't face sex and is thinking of adopting.

An episiotomy, as we have seen in Chapter 4, is deliberate surgical injury to the most sensitive part of a woman's body. It is sometimes necessary in order to get a baby out fast and start it breathing or because it seems that without an incision there may be a tear into the rectum. Even so, most tears into the rectum – third-degree tears – occur as an extension of an episiotomy, and are the result of being cut.[147]

I. D. Graham, in his book *Episiotomy: Challenging Obstetric Interventions*, says:

> *This so called 'trivial' operation should be an important public health issue as it is the most frequently performed surgical procedure, after cutting the umbilical cord, and is not without sometimes serious side effects. It is performed on millions of women annually ... Where only 28 per cent of women giving birth vaginally in Belgium received the operation, close to 100 per cent of Japanese women and women in Central and Eastern Europe having vaginal deliveries experience an episiotomy ... The haphazard way that national statistics on episiotomy use are often collected and reported, if they happen to be collected and reported at all, is an indication of just how widely accepted the operation is in many countries and the lack of significance that has been placed on it by health officials.[148]*

133

A woman who has had an episiotomy may be out of pain two to three weeks after the birth. But this is unusual. She is more likely to still have pain for two to three months afterwards when intercourse is attempted.

On the other hand, a woman who has had a small tear or has an intact perineum feels bruised and tender in the days immediately after birth, but by two to three weeks this has passed.

When in the early 1980s I decided to investigate the experience of episiotomy and suturing of the perineum, surgery which over 70 per cent of women having their first babies and 38 per cent of those having subsequent babies underwent, astonishingly no research had been done to find out what women thought about it. There had been research on the angle of the incision and the material to use for sutures but none investigating women's experiences of being cut and sewn up again. The information I received from women led me to conclude that episiotomy was our western way of female genital mutilation.

We know now that a tear – unless it is a very large one – heals more easily than an episiotomy and causes far less pain. Much depends on the skill with which the wound is repaired. It is not necessary to suture a small tear. It will heal better naturally.

It has also been discovered that injury to the perineum has to do with the conduct of delivery. If a woman is urged to push without discretion, or a baby is pulled out fast, there is almost bound to be perineal damage. When a woman is able to 'breathe out' her baby and the delivery is not hurried, perineal tissues can usually fan out and the birth is a smooth passage. A good midwife has the skills to retain the integrity of a woman's perineum whenever possible, even with a big baby. This is not a matter of sleight of hand. She may not guard the perineum at all. She may not touch the baby's head as it slides over the perineum. It is largely to do with her relationship with the mother, how she nurtures her self-confidence – and the way both women work in harmony with the power generated in the female body and the descent and spontaneous beautiful rotation of the baby's head.

Concern about changes in the vagina and perineum and to muscles deep inside is a recurrent theme in anxiety after childbirth. A woman who has had an episiotomy often feels that she is a stranger to her own body, and after being poked, prodded, stretched, lacerated and sewn up she may be afraid to look at or touch her genitals and feel, justifiably, mutilated. If she did not have an episiotomy but believes she should have, she may imagine her vagina as a gaping hole, a sagging mess of ragged tissues, or, in contrast, if she has been sutured, tight as a pea pod that may pop open if touched.

One woman who rang me in distress had a tear that was not sutured but had wanted an episiotomy, was worried that her uterus was falling out and could not accept reassurance from the obstetrician. She was doing pelvic floor exercises and the physiotherapist said her muscles were strong. Unfortunately a midwife who had a young baby herself and suffered similar anxiety commented unwisely, 'I know. And after you have a bath or swim a cup of water falls out.' As a result she dared not go swimming and had stopped having baths because of her fear of infection. In fact, water cannot collect in the vagina.

Immediately after birth post-partum bleeding may last three to four weeks – sometimes shorter, sometimes longer – with the blood gradually changing from red to pink. At first it is like having a heavy period. Pads stick to skin that is bruised and may also have been nicked, and the whole area is exquisitely tender if pubic hair was shaved and is starting to grow again. A woman's perineum is hot, aching and swollen. Sitting is uncomfortable and after stitches it feels as if she is sitting on jagged glass. She cannot wear jeans because they rub, and constant bleeding makes her feel dirty and smelly.

Women usually tolerate this for a few weeks. They think it is part of the price they pay for having the baby. But they become distressed when it goes on and on and on, when any lovemaking that involves the vagina is impossible, and they have urinary incontinence and sometimes faecal incontinence, too.

A woman whose child is now two years old described what she went through and what she feels now:

> They decided on a trial of forceps. I told them, 'Please try and tell me what is going on.' The man who seemed to be in charge said, 'Are you a doctor? Mind your own business!' I felt like I was being attacked.
>
> I went to my GP afterwards because I needed to talk about it. I felt I had been assaulted. And I was still so sore down there making love was out of the question. He told me I had psycho-sexual problems and that I was depressed. I said, 'I am not depressed. I am bloody mad!'
>
> I don't know where to turn for help.

The shape of the vagina always changes with childbirth. Some women are shocked and disturbed by this because they did not expect it. Even when they have not had an episiotomy, they feel 'deformed' and want to return to 'normal'. Women often never see other women's genitals, so we have no idea of the variety of shapes there are, like different orchids – some small, others large, some neat, some voluptuously complicated. After giving birth the outer tissues of the vagina are flexible and more open, like a flower in full bloom, compared with the tight rosebud shape that a girl of 12 may have.

Some women go to great lengths to restructure their genitals, choosing laser vaginal 'rejuvenation' and resculpting or, more popularly, a 'fanny tuck'. In the US this is said to be the fastest growing area of plastic surgery. 'Make it like I never had children, like I'm 16 again', one cosmetic surgeon says he was told by a patient.[149] 'Designer vaginas' are not that different from the ritual female genital mutilation practised over large parts of Africa. In each case women are led to believe that a narrow, tight vagina is attractive and preferred by men.

After a straightforward birth it is normal for the tissues of the perineum to be bruised for a week or so. When a woman passes urine it may sting as it goes over surface abrasions, but they soon heal. If she has had an episiotomy and/or large tear that has been sutured, there is a line of stitches rather like a zip and a very tender bump at the base of the vagina, between it and the anus, or slightly to one side, or even if it does not hurt, a knob of scar tissue that feels stiff: 'It feels as if I have a tampon half in, half out.' 'It's like a zip inside.' Because nerves have been cut, there may be an area where she feels numb. This is especially likely if she has had an episiotomy that extended into a tear. If she had a first-degree or second-degree tear, which may not even have needed suturing, she is more or less the same shape as before, but there are extra creases in the tissues and some frilly edges. Massage with a vegetable oil or nut oil helps relieve the stiffness and tenderness and enables her to feel she is in touch with her body again.

If her vagina is very tight following suturing of an episiotomy, she may be anxious that she is going to split during sexual intercourse. This can make her tighten up involuntary. It can be so severe that she has vaginismus and her partner cannot enter. Once this happens the experience sets the scene for further dyspareunia (painful sex). She can help herself if she introduces first one finger, then two, then – when she feels ready for it – three, while releasing the muscles around her lower vagina.

Genital repair surgery can be performed if a woman is too tight for intercourse or in pain. It can also be used to correct bladder and bowel dysfunction, but it may be wise to wait some months, since hormone changes in the first year after birth can soothe and mend sensitive tissues, and pelvic floor exercises done every day help re-tone muscles. Sometimes full tissue flexibility is restored when a woman is no longer lactating.

Some women (after 0.5 to 2 per cent of vaginal births) have partial or complete rupture of the anal sphincter muscle – a third-degree tear. This can cause great distress. They find it difficult to get accurate information and feel very isolated. Their partners may also be anxious and express this by not wanting to discuss the subject. Healing takes place gradually over the next few years. But meanwhile women may suffer from faecal incontinence, urgency, perineal pain and pain with intercourse, even after a primary repair operation. There is urgent need for systematic counselling and follow-up from members of a dedicated team who are supportive and really know what they are talking about.[150,151]

RECLAIMING YOUR GENITALS

If you are anxious about your perineum and vagina, have a look in the mirror. Feel around with your fingertips to discover the geography of sensation – any parts that hurt, parts that are numb, parts where touch feels good. It is important to discover this and to communicate it to your partner.

Explore sensation in this way *before* seeking advice from a doctor. You need to have all the information you can get if you decide to seek medical help. *You know your body best.*

One way to check if your pelvic floor muscles are well toned is to interrupt a stream of urine. If you can do this, they are in good condition. Remember to finish the investigation by releasing them again to empty your bladder.

Any muscles atrophy if not used. Muscles around the vagina, bladder and rectum need to be mobilised if they are to recover tone. If we went round with slack facial muscles and rarely talked or chewed food, our mouths would hang open in a way similar to that of many women's genital muscles after childbirth. This may become worse as muscles get older. It is not only the fear that mobilising them will cause pain that stops some women exercising these muscles – often women detach themselves from this part of the body because of a traumatic delivery and an episiotomy.

When we talk and eat, and when facial expressions change, we tone muscles. Pelvic floor muscles need to be exercised in a similar way. They need to be toned. But a smash and grab raid on the pelvic floor does not work. There is a more subtle approach. We can 'talk' with these muscles:

- 'Talking'. A good time is when you are sitting down and on the telephone or at the computer. Feel the muscles working against the chair. Exaggerate pelvic floor 'pronunciation' for the greatest effect. Do not contract the buttock muscles (glutei) or the inside thigh muscles (adductors). Doing that may mask the fact that the pelvic floor muscles are not really working. Avoid tightening pelvic floor muscles so hard that they start to tremble. A muscle quivers when it is not strong enough to cope with a sustained contraction. So take it gently, starting with light, short movements and building up activity gradually. When a muscle is contracted tightly the flow of blood through it is reduced, and hence the oxygen. When the contraction is released blood flows through freely. So alternate contraction and release in a dance-like movement increases the oxygen supply to the muscles and avoids strain.

- The Cherry. Think of a small soft fruit – a cherry, perhaps – inside the circle of muscles around the vagina and imagine that you are chewing and eating it. As you 'swallow' the fruit, feel the muscles being pulled up towards your uterus. Rest for a few seconds and then 'eat' another piece of fruit.

- The Peach. Think of a much larger soft fruit – an apricot or peach, perhaps – with a smooth, velvety skin. 'Scan' the curved surface of this fruit with your pelvic muscles, using a sweeping, stroking movement. Then imagine the fruit crushed and the juices flowing out of it. Slowly, deliberately, suck in the juice with your pelvic floor muscles. Then rest. Now scan again, suck in and swallow. With these last two exercises you will contract not only the muscles of the vagina but those that encircle the rectum, anus and urethra. All these muscles work in a co-ordinated way with each other.

- Pelvic rock. As your pelvic floor is contracted you tend to rock your pelvis forward; press down the small of your back and tighten the trans-abdominal muscles. The result is a dance-like pelvic rock.

An American gynaecologist – Dr Kegel – was the first to introduce to the western world the idea of exercising the pelvic floor muscles.

Women had been doing it in Japan and other parts of the east for centuries. As a result the pelvic floor became known as the 'Kegel muscle' and the exercise as 'Kegels'. In the US women who attended childbirth classes often had stickers saying 'Kegel', which they stuck on their fridge doors to remind them to exercise. A problem with Kegels is that they can become an attack on the pelvic floor and cause strain. It is clear that this is happening if the muscles start to tremble. I also don't like the idea of labelling any part of a woman's body with a gynaecologist's name. It is not his. It's mine! So here is my version of an all-round exercise for toning pelvic floor muscles:

• The Lift. Think of the muscles as a lift in a building with five floors. Gradually tighten them to make the lift go up from the ground to the first floor, to the second floor, third floor, by which time you will feel pressure on your bladder, the fourth floor and then the fifth floor. Be careful to go on breathing as you do this, and don't attempt to pull your muscles up with your shoulders. Hold the contraction for four or five seconds and then gently descend to the ground floor. Finish by going back up to the first floor so that you end with a toning action. This is a good exercise to do while waiting at the supermarket checkout or for traffic lights to change. Link it with things you do every day so that you can increase pelvic floor vitality by mobilising the muscles regularly.

• The Smile. When a woman is depressed her pelvic floor muscles tend to sag. When she feels positive and alert they are naturally toned. Greet every morning with a pelvic floor 'smile', and whenever you feel under pressure or that it is a drag to get through the day take the opportunity to give a big pelvic floor smile. It may make you feel much better!

SEXUAL DIFFICULTIES

Sexual problems described by distressed women are usually associated with episiotomy in which accidental injury occurred – a tear extending into the rectum, for example – clumsy suturing, and occasionally massive haemorrhage after a vein has been sliced through by mistake.

We may infer from the ways in which some doctors justify routine episiotomy that they are unaware of research evidence concerning the risks and benefits of this surgery. A woman whose baby was a year old told me that she is unable to have penetrative sex because of a rigid scar. She had an operation to repair this, but it failed. She said:

> *The doctor told me, 'Every fair haired woman will need an episiotomy, whereas black ladies don't', and he turned to my daughter who was about 10 months and said, 'Of course, she'll be the same', at which I nearly punched him.*

A woman rang me about her faecal incontinence, which dates from 20 years ago when she delivered her first child by forceps. She had an episiotomy and the wound became infected. 'My bottom was facing the doors where everyone passing could see it. It was the first delivery the doctor had done. He swore at me when my legs jerked in stirrups.' Her son knows that his birth caused her incontinence, and feels bad about it.

However, sexual problems are often more complex and need to be considered in a psycho-social context. A woman whose episiotomy was sutured too tightly said, 'It has made me a virgin again. The wound also became infected.' They are Catholic and do not practise contraception. Intercourse is painful, and she is terrified of getting pregnant again because of her traumatic birth experience.

Sex after a traumatic birth

- The first few times a couple make love – and sometimes for much longer – they should do so without penetration.
- Full intercourse should not take place until bleeding has stopped. Bleeding is a sign that there are still raw patches in the endometrium (the lining of the uterus) and these are vulnerable to infection.
- Gentle finger-tip touches are a vital part of lovemaking.
- A partner should never enter until a woman is aroused, and her spontaneous lubrication is evidence of this.
- If you would like your partner to penetrate, it is important to leave the action, and all thrusting, to you, as only you can tell what you can take, what movements are pleasurable and which are painful.
- Make love *after* you have fed and settled the baby. You are less likely to be interrupted and your breasts will be less tender. In the first few months it may be difficult to find a gap when you are not needed and when you are readily aroused. You may be so relieved that at last the baby is sleeping that you want only to sleep yourself. This is normal.

- Desire fluctuates. On a high immediately after a good birth, you may long for sex in a few days or weeks. As parenting demands your energy and concentration, you may not be able to give much attention to sex, and it becomes brief and spasmodic. This is normal, too!
- Following a traumatic birth you may feel you never want to make love ever again, and the thought of possibly getting pregnant fills you with dread. That is understandable. Give yourself time. Find other ways of showing your love. You are unlikely to get pregnant while you are fully breastfeeding. Once you start to give any other kind of milk, or solids, there is a chance of conception, since ovulation is likely to occur a couple of weeks *before* your first period.
- If you decide to use a condom, do so with lashings of lubricant gel.

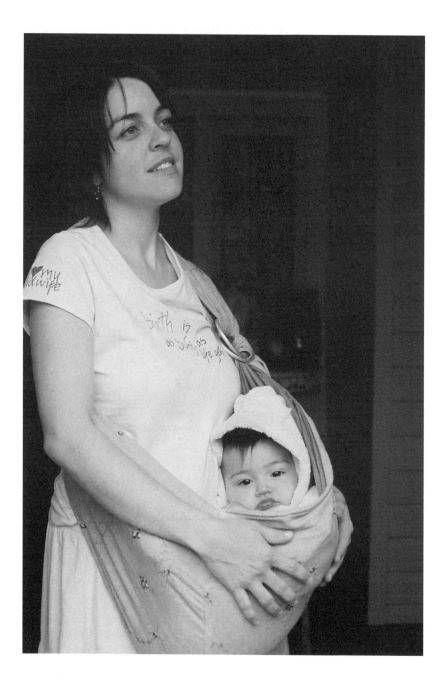

12

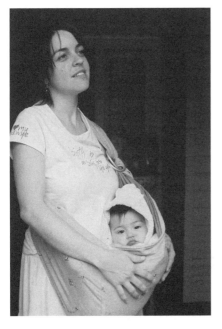

HERE ARE SUGGESTIONS so that you can work out your own strategy – not advice. You will know yourself what you have the courage to face now. Telling the story of a distressing birth is an important element in healing.

PUT YOUR BIRTH STORY INTO WORDS

Difficult as it is to face up to a distressing birth experience, it is important to examine it closely and all the feelings it aroused.

Research into women's recall of their first birth experiences some 20 years later reveals that memories remain vivid and powerful.

> *After it is over, women often need to talk about the labor, ponder it, mull it over, and make sense of it. They have to put into words what they felt. For them labor was not experienced at a verbal or cognitive level. They have to match what happened on the inside (the inner reality) with what 'really happened' (the outer reality) as represented by what others saw. This process of integrating and understanding these various parts takes time and effort.*[152]

GET HOLD OF YOUR RECORDS

It is not good enough to be shown your notes only to have them whipped away at the end of a Birth Afterthoughts or counselling session. You need to hang on to them. If necessary, make a copy.

They way the professionals who cared for you saw your labour and birth is likely to be very different from how you remember it. An intense personal experience will have little resemblance to medical notes and a partogram. You may have forgotten or never really taken on board some things that were said or happened. The records may have omitted important events, or events may have been recorded incorrectly, or sometimes you can see that information has been altered.

If you do not have your notes, ring the records office at the hospital where you gave birth, the head of midwifery or, if you had a birth centre or home birth, the midwife who attended you, and say that you would like the case notes to put with your birth story so that you have a full record of your baby's birth. The Association for Improvements in the Maternity Services (AIMS) can advise you how to do this and what you should bear in mind. For more information see 'Useful addresses' (pp. 169–73).

Go through the notes with whoever was your birth companion and also, if possible, with the midwife. Jot down your observations about any discrepancies and omissions. This will be useful in piecing together your own narrative of the birth. Once you have a framework you can add information about the emotional impact of each event.

This is likely to be very painful for you. Don't try to do it alone. If possible, fill in the blanks and discuss the options that your caregivers had and what they did and said, and how you reacted, with your antenatal teacher, someone who is giving you post-natal support, or a trusted friend who understands about birth.

How to crack the code

There will probably be a graph of an 'ideal labour' stretching in a steep line from the bottom left corner on the chart to the top right. This indicates dilatation of the cervix. The time is shown on the left side. There will be another line recording how your cervix dilated – or failed to dilate – with crosses on it to indicate observations and interventions. These are coded and abbreviated.

On the page before the graph there will be notes about your pregnancy. Look especially at those for the last week. (See Table on pp. 146–7.)

A SELF-HELP GROUP

One way to try to come to terms with a traumatic birth might be through a self-help group – going into an email chat room, perhaps, hearing about other women's distressing experiences and sharing ideas so that you are less isolated. On the other hand, you may hear repeated accounts of atrocity as members tell of medical misman-agement and personal misery. Unless it leads to action, it does nothing to change the situation. They are recycling their pain.

Women's self-help groups grew out of the feminist movement. From a basis of shared experience they challenged powerful social systems that thrive on gender inequalities. This is what happened with the growth and globalisation of the Boston Women's Health Collective, now renamed Our Bodies, Our Selves.

A self-help group may feed on itself and its members' unhappi-ness without making the move into politics. Verta Taylor, a feminist sociologist, writes: 'As might be expected, self-help displays some of the same qualities of the modern institutions that it challenges, namely a heightened emphasis on the interests of the individual rather than community. . . .' She observes that in sharing anger, anxiety, depression and guilt and seeking medical and psychiatric solutions women define their problems in medical terms. Though she is writing about post-natal depression, it is clear from some of the examples she cites that women had multiple interventions and probably experienced post-traumatic stress disorder as much as, or rather than, depression.[153]

DECODING YOUR CASE NOTES

Before labour

LMP	Last Menstrual Period
EDD	Estimated Date of Delivery
FH	Fetal Heart
FHH	Fetal Heart Heard
FHNH	Fetal Heart Not Heard
FMH	Fetal Movement Felt
FMNF	Fetal Movement Not Felt
NAD/NIL	No abnormality detected
PROT	Protein in urine, usually recorded as −, tr (trace), +, ++, +++
OED	Oedema. May be recorded as swelling
BP	Blood Pressure
↑ BP	Hypertension − raised blood pressure
PET	Pre-eclampsia − a condition specific to pregnancy with raised blood pressure, proteinuria and degrees of systemic dysfunction
BR	Breech − baby is coming out bottom or feet first
Transverse	The baby is lying across your uterus
CEPH	Cephalic (head down)
VX	Vertex (head down)
E or ENG	Engaged (baby's head down in your pelvis ready for birth)
NE	Not Engaged − the leading part of the baby has not yet entered the main part of the pelvis
A fraction, e.g. 5/5	An estimate of how deeply the baby's head has descended into your pelvis. May be recorded 5/5 ↑ (high, not fixed into the pelvic brim yet) or 5/5 ((well engaged in the pelvis)
PP	Placenta Praevia (the placenta is low lying in the uterus to a lesser or greater extent)
PROM	Premature or pre-labour Rupture of Membranes (often used indiscriminately)
SFD	Small for Dates
LFD	Large for Dates (both these are often inaccurate estimates)
GTT	Glucose Tolerance Test (to diagnose diabetes of pregnancy)

HB	Haemoglobin level (to test for anaemia)
FH	Fundal height: measuring the height of the top of your uterus indicates how well your baby is growing, usually recorded as FH = 32/40 or FH = 32 weeks
↓ liquor	Reduced amount of amniotic fluid (oligohydramnios) (on estimate)
↑ liquor	Increased amount of amniotic fluid (polyhydramnios) (on estimate)

During labour

NIEL	Not in Established Labour
EL	Early Labour
VE	Vaginal Examination
LOA	Left Occipito Anterior (the baby is lying on your left facing your back, a very good position)
ROA	Right Occipito Anterior (the baby is lying on your right facing your back, a very good position)
LOP	Left Occipito Posterior (the baby is lying on your left facing your front)
ROP	Right Occipito Posterior (the baby is lying on your right facing your front)
LOL	Left Occipito Lateral (the baby is lying on your left with an ear towards the front)
ROL	Right Occipito Lateral (the baby is lying on your right with an ear towards the front)
ROL	The baby is lying across your uterus
Memb Intact	Intact Membranes (waters have not broken)
SROM	Spontaneous Rupture of Membranes
ARM	Artificial Rupture of Membranes
IOL	Induction of Labour – intervention to stimulate uterine contractions before the onset of spontaneous labour
Sp Lab	Spontaneous Labour
Aug	Augmentation of Labour – intervention to speed up labour
Mec liquor	Meconium stained liquor (baby has had first bowel motion before birth)

147

Either way, the mental illness she described was clearly not due to endocrine factors or simply to having no social support post-partum. It was associated with the mechanistic and technocratic management of childbirth and specific practices that deny women autonomy and result in them being distressed, anxious and having nightmares and panic attacks.

When individuals join together to form pressure groups, that is political action. Yet if the care they seek is to demand more medical interventions, claiming that women have a 'right' to epidurals and pain-free birth or to choose a Caesarean section to escape having to go through vaginal birth, they willingly surrender control to the medical system. Members of the group may see epidurals and Caesarean sections on demand as a simple solution to their distress, thinking that this will ensure a birth without pain and that they will be in control.

Demanding twilight sleep: control or subservience?

This has happened before with the introduction of 'twilight sleep' – a mix of scopolamine and morphine – in the US in the first half of the twentieth century. Obstetricians were not insisting on its use. Women were. An article was published in *McClure's Magazine* describing a method of painless birth invented in Germany, and a strong women's movement quickly grew to promote it. Doctors acceded to powerful pressure from patients who in a highly competitive market could pay for what they wanted. An obstetrician who would not provide twilight sleep was likely to go out of business and be left only with non-paying clinic patients.

This 'pain-free' birth was bought at a price. The effects of twilight sleep were horrendous. Though they could remember nothing of the birth or how they behaved, women became like wild animals in a trap. 'Scoped' patients threw themselves about, screamed, swore and growled. The noises issuing from labour rooms came as if from a hellhole. They were put in high, barred and padded cots with a sheet over the top and down the sides so that they could not escape or injure themselves. These drugs were passed through the bloodstream to their babies, too. In attempting to gain control, women surrendered control completely.

The pressure group for twilight sleep held public demonstrations on the streets and in large stores. It accused the medical profession of denying women a basic right of pain-free childbirth. Only when in 1915 Mrs Carmody – the charismatic leader of the movement –

died in childbirth, did doubts about the safety of this drug cocktail prevail over the enthusiasm.

Meanwhile many doctors had given in to women's demands, because once their patients were under the influence of twilight sleep they could busy themselves with other things without needing to worry about the doctor–patient relationship or adopting a bedside manner. Twilight sleep activism waned, but the drug was by then firmly established in practice and remained in use throughout the twentieth century.

Women's struggle to have control over birth resulted in the medical system gaining more control. 'Ironically, the twilight sleep movement helped change the definition of birthing from a natural home event ... to an illness requiring hospitalisation. ...'[154] It provides a historic precedent for epidurals and Caesarean sections on demand.

FACE UP TO FEAR

You do not get rid of fear by asserting that it is groundless – however many times the statement is repeated. An approach to fear based on facile and misleading reassurance is worse than useless. Nor should fear be replaced by gratitude because everything is done for the baby's sake. Articles sometimes appear in women's magazines that unequivocally accept midwifery and obstetric interventions, and treat each instrumental and Caesarean delivery as if it should be welcomed because it is a matter of urgency to avoid the death of the baby.

In attempting to reassure, books may mislead, too. A book that aims to offer 'wisdom and reassurance' heads a section on Caesareans with 'Fear Fact' and goes on to say, 'The odds are against it, but even if you have one, it won't be unnecessary, and you'll recover well.' That is nonsense. The advice to the reader is:

> We must try to think and act like good mothers. What would a good mother say to her daughter if she had to have a c-section? She'd tell her that the goal in all of this was to end the day with a healthy baby and a healthy mom.[155]

Unfortunately, this is what a fearful pregnant woman is being told all the time by family, friends, casual acquaintances and professionals. She probably already feels guilty and 'unnatural', and this only makes it worse. Health is not only a matter of the absence of physical disability; it is about emotional well-being, too.

149

TELL THE STORY

To really understand any experience it has to be perceived in its entirety and looked at from different angles like a scene being described. If we are too close or ourselves part of it, we can present only fragments. The best view of the valley may be from the hills, and of a mountain range from the plain below.

An important part of understanding a traumatic birth is creating a narrative that shapes and frames it. Women struggle to do this without needing to be told. But the stories are often interrupted, denied, interpreted and resisted by listeners who are made uncomfortable by the telling or want to remodel it from their own angle. Very few people seem able to sit and listen to a woman's story without intervening. They may treat it as a fragment of her imagination, explaining the trauma in terms of her anxiety or mental instability. Numerous papers have been published about post-natal depression, for example, that ascribe it to the woman's own faulty ways of thinking and feeling. Studies examine psychiatric patients who are suffering this distress by searching for the cause inside the woman and predicting those who will have post-natal depression.

A new illness has been invented – tokophobia, a morbid fear of birth. Articles about it have even appeared in parenting magazines. 'Primary tokophobia' is dread of birth that exists before pregnancy. 'Secondary tokophobia' is pregnancy fear after a previous traumatic birth.[156] So along with agoraphobia (open spaces), claustrophobia (closed spaces), hydrophobia (water) and arachnophobia (spiders) there is now tokophobia. It may be discussed as if it were an internally generated psychiatric illness rather than in terms of how women are treated in birth. It is removed from its social context and ignores issues of power and powerlessness – what happens when individuals are fed into and processed through medical institutions like car parts on a conveyor belt.

It is easy for a health professional to feel personally threatened and accused by the birth account a woman offers and to attempt to justify actions as necessary for safety, and to loyally defend hospital policy and personnel.

THE LISTENING EXPERIENCE

To listen may sound easy. It isn't. A listener is not just an automatic recording machine. It entails giving yourself, opening, being aware – and demands stamina, too! The listener needs to be in focus and, in the way the philosopher Martin Buber described, create a quality of personal relationship in which the woman is not 'you' but 'thou'.[157] There are times when one distressed woman after another talks to me about her suffering and I feel emotionally shredded. I need to enter a quiet space inside myself, and I do this even when I am busy with tasks that have to be completed and when everything seems to be rushing around me.

This is 'centring down', a kind of inner solitude that I learned in Quaker meetings. Others may call it prayer, relaxation, meditation or simply 'standing back' or 'switching off'. But the point is that I cannot ditch the distress that these women have trusted me with, yet it no longer weighs me down and exhausts me.

As you listen, do not seek solutions. Just wait in silence. You will gain strength and greater understanding.

When a woman appeals for help, it is easy to be drawn into judgement and offer advice, pulled into the arena of conflict. Instead, help her to explore possible ways forward. This is how I empower her.

On the phone

There are bound to be times when a woman calls you and says, 'I was the one who had a Caesarean last year.' She might be one of 20 or 30 women who had Caesareans whom you have talked to recently. She has bared her soul to you and expects you to remember the baby's name and you don't even know whether it was a boy or a girl and how many children she has already.

I have learned that it is best to be honest and say, 'You'll have to fill me in with more details.' Sometimes I recollect her voice and say so. Or something she says offers a clue to her story. Then I pick up on that. I have come to realise that I do not need to be superhuman or have a fantastic memory. I think it is probably more important to stay in the moment for the woman and focus on what she is saying now than to be able to produce evidence of all that she has told you in a previous call. So I ask questions again.

A caller who pictures you sitting behind a desk with headphones at a call centre will get rather a shock when you say, 'Hang on a minute. I have to take something out of the oven.' Or 'I have two children in the room with me and we're painting. Give me a moment and I'll go to another phone.' 'Oh, my three-year-old has fallen down. Just a minute!' Or 'I apologise for the banging. The builders are in.' But it is better to do this than to try to cope with the inevitable interruptions.

It is always OK to say you're going to a quiet room or to your desk, and to pick up the extension there. The problem is that if there is a festive meal going on in the room where you originally answered the phone, no one may remember to replace the receiver and your conversation will be interrupted by gales of laughter and your shouts from the other end of the house, 'Put the phone back on!' At least when they at last do this the woman to whom you are talking realises that the conversation is private.

The help that can be given is more than just sitting and listening. It is listening, soaking up – and then reflecting back. It is both acceptance and, through reflecting back, validating the story and revealing it with greater clarity. For a woman who is confused, and in a tangle of emotions, this starts the process of unravelling. It is not something that is done *for* her. It is something that *she* does. The listener may ask some questions as she tells the story, enabling both to make more sense of what happened. These might be: 'What do you think was in your midwife's mind?', 'Why do you think the obstetrician did that?', 'Looking back at it, how do you think your partner was feeling then?' or 'When that was done how did you feel? What did you do?' 'How did they react? Why do you think that was?'. Sometimes, when a woman has been trying to present an unemotional catalogue of events, this opens the door for the expression of strong emotions.

Some psychiatrists are critical of any attempts at therapy that encourage focus on the trauma. They see it as potentially harmful because it re-exposes the person who suffers from post-traumatic stress disorder to the traumatic events. They claim that it encourages 'preoccupation with the past, a victim mindset, and erosion of the sense of personal agency and confidence. ... This professionally directed attention to the past, and to "emotion" can become fundamentally anti-therapeutic.'[158]

This is an issue that needs addressing. But perhaps the key in that statement is the phrase 'professionally directed attention'. A woman who is distressed after childbirth is not being forced to confront the trauma. The fact is that she cannot get away from it. It is going round and round in her head all the time. It is haunting her. Other people keep on telling her to forget it or deny that the experience could possibly have been as she says it was. Or they say it 'had to be like that, for the baby's sake'. Now someone listens to her who accepts her story and all the emotion that comes with it, does not trivialise it, nor try to hurry her on, is not frightened by it, waits patiently as she cries, and treats her as a reasonable human being.

I believe that when a woman is distressed after childbirth she benefits from both exploring the traumatic experience and also from looking ahead. She is helped to move forward into the future, and to do this she has to find strength within herself. Before that can happen she needs to create a narrative of the traumatic experience and have it validated. It cannot be swept into oblivion. So ways have to be found of enabling her to stand back and look at it carefully – what happened between individuals involved and the emotional impact on her at the time and after. Only then can she move on. Eventually, like poetry, the narrative of the trauma that she creates is 'emotion recollected in tranquillity'.[159]

The building of a therapeutic narrative may be easier if a woman tells the story as if it happened to someone else, and might be an article in a magazine. It enables her to view the trauma from greater distance. Or she may want to draw or paint a scene from the birth or the recurring image that tortures her.

A woman may try to make sense of her experience by pointing to elements in the pregnancy and birth that in themselves do not explain or justify the interventions to which she was subjected. It is important not to endorse obstetric actions that, in retrospect, were not based on research evidence and were probably unnecessary. This happens when she says that she had an induction or a planned Caesarean section, for example, 'because it was a big baby', 'I'd gone a week overdue', 'I'm only 5 feet 4 inches', 'I'm 38 and it was my first', or 'my last baby was a Caesarean delivery'.

Yet it is vital that the listener does not get drawn into arguments. Ask gentle questions. Ask searching questions. But don't get into a 'yes, but' situation. The listener's task is to hear what the woman is saying, reflect back, and help *her* reflect back – not to superimpose another authority.

Reflective listening isn't about 'communication skills'. It is nothing to do with techniques. It comes from respecting the other person, hearing what they *are* saying, and *not* saying, and never passing judgement on them.

In any conversation, whether it aims to be therapeutic or not, one participant may attempt to superimpose authority, sum up their own opinions or push the other person into coming to a conclusion.

If I am tempted to put pressure on a woman to take action, I hold back and wait patiently, with sounds that signify interest, concern, understanding and sympathy, and sometimes doubt, questioning or surprise. This will often be enough to give her the support she needs to tell, and to think through, her story, and even to go on from there to develop a strategy for a subsequent pregnancy and birth.

In some cases distressed women have confronted the possibility of death in childbirth – from pre-eclampsia, haemorrhage or liver disease, for example, and are still overwhelmed by the feeling that they are dying. They have panic attacks in which they cannot breathe, and are jolted awake from nightmares of death and dying. Because life-threatening illness is rare in childbirth in northern industrial countries today it is all the more shocking when it could be a reality. A woman may have wanted a home birth, made a carefully thought-out birth plan, for example, and suddenly all control is taken from her and she witnesses caregivers panicking around her.

After the birth it may be hard for her to get other people to under-stand the urgency of that threat because it is beyond their experience. I realise that sometimes when I listen on the phone to women's accounts of these potential disasters I half withdraw, not quite sure whether I believe their exact version of events. When I do this I fail to validate the intensity of their feelings and the emotional impact of a near-death experience.

How do you deal with your own grief when you listen to a distressing account? I know that tears come into my eyes and I sniff, and I may moan as well. The other person hears this, of course. It is nothing you need be ashamed of. Apologise if you want to and say, 'I do find what you're telling me so awful!' or something like that. There are times when you are drawn into the story through empathy and compassion. That is just as it should be.

As I come close to ending a conversation I aim to do four things: to finish on a positive note, increase a woman's self-confidence, confirm with her some action she can take (if she feels strong enough) that will help her move forward and let her know that I am keen to learn what happens and to hear from her again. This springs from my spontaneous interest in her as a unique individual.

I see each conversation as a bridge between us both, and also a bridge to the future.

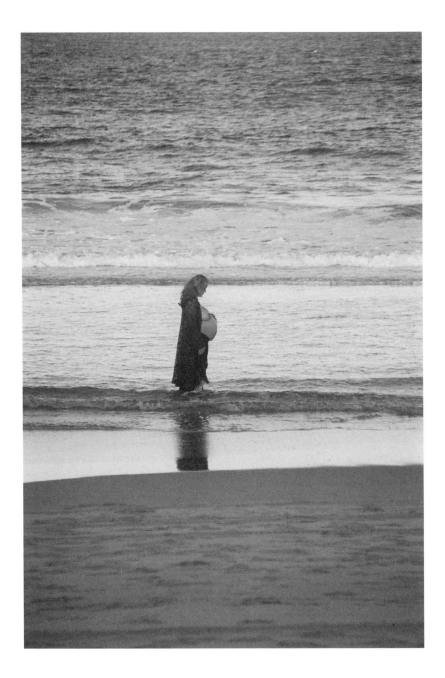

PREGNANT AGAIN

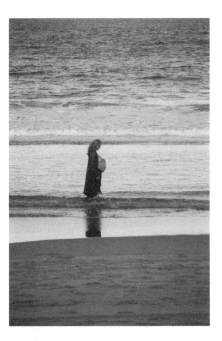

MANY WOMEN FACE A CRISIS when they find themselves pregnant again. They may panic when even contemplating a
pregnancy. One thing to do is to plan ahead to make this birth
as different as possible from the last. It is usually wise to switch to
a different hospital, or from obstetrician to midwife care, to seek a
one-to-one relationship with the midwife and, if this is unlikely to
be a high-risk birth, to consider a birth centre or home birth. If you
have a chance to do so, shop around. This is your body, your baby
and your birth.

A PLANNED CAESAREAN

An elective Caesarean is often misrepresented as being 'too posh to push' when, in fact, a woman is anxious and afraid. This may be the result of a traumatic previous birth with induction, severe pain, care from strangers who were anonymous and constantly changing, instrumental delivery or, perhaps, an emergency Caesarean.

It may also be because of the mistaken belief that Caesareans are safer. One private hospital in London charges £600 extra for a 'no indicated risk' Caesarean. Susan Bewley and Jayne Cockburn, consultant obstetricians at Guy's and St Thomas's and Frimley Park, comment that this could be a coded way to say, 'Have second thoughts about treading this path', but may 'make women think celebrities and those who can afford it are buying something better than is otherwise rationed on the NHS!'[160]

An obstetrician who agrees to a request for or encourages an elective Caesarean is, according to these obstetric specialists, not only performing unnecessary surgery, but failing to deal with a woman's fear and anxiety. 'The implicit message of Caesarean section "on request" . . . is that it must be better, thus reinforcing cultural apprehensions.' Choices in childbirth are not just a matter of spreading a display of vendibles in front of a patient and saying, 'Go ahead and choose; it's your life.' This is malpractice.[161] The language of choice is used as rhetoric to suggest that all options are equal and persuade women that decisions about birth are no different from selecting dishes from an à la carte menu. An elective Caesarean gives them the illusion of control. 'The danger in not recognising fears and phobia but renaming them "requests" or even "rights" is that they remain unaddressed and reinforced.'[162]

These obstetricians analyse what they call 'morbidity of mythological proportions' about vaginal birth and the belief that it inevitably damages the pelvic floor and makes women incontinent of urine, and that a Caesarean prevents this. It doesn't. It is pregnancy, particularly if a woman is overweight, that does it. And it can nearly always be treated.

Bladder and bowel problems and pelvic floor dysfunction may occur after a Caesarean birth, too. Sometimes an obstetrician suggests to a woman that a Caesarean with another pregnancy will provide the answer to difficulties she has had after a previous vaginal birth. Unfortunately, this is not the case. A study of pelvic floor dysfunction after 80 elective and 104 emergency Caesareans compared with 100 non-instrumental vaginal births showed that after a Caesarean women had just as many pelvic floor symptoms.[163]

Vaginal birth does not have to be violent. It can be gentle. Instead of choosing a Caesarean, it makes sense to examine why the previous delivery caused such damage and see how in another birth a woman can, with caregivers tuned to her needs and not rushing the delivery, work *with* her body instead of injuring it.

If a woman is terrified of birth, surgery may not provide a solution. A better way is to explore her options and examine exactly what she is afraid of.

VBAC (VAGINAL BIRTH AFTER CAESAREAN)

Women who ring the Birth Crisis line to talk about a traumatic birth have often had a Caesarean section and dread being compelled to have one next time.

If the same conditions do not recur in the next pregnancy, there is probably no good reason to have surgery. Instead, it can be a VBAC. Obstetricians sometimes call this 'a trial of labour' or 'trial of scar'. But that is bound to make a woman doubt that it can succeed. It is a term redolent of witch-ducking and other forms of torture in medieval times.

In the US it has become increasingly difficult to get a VBAC, let alone an HBAC (home birth after Caesarean). Insurance companies will not provide care for hospital personnel unless they have a team ready for a crash Caesarean available at all times and able to spring into action. This means that women have to move perhaps 200 miles to a large medical centre with all the facilities, or risk out-of-hospital birth without adequate support, if they are determined to have a VBAC. Realistic choices are denied them.

A woman's commitment to and confidence in giving birth vaginally after a previous Caesarean contributes strongly to the likelihood of success.[164] When this is undermined the risk of a repeat Caesarean is increased. She needs support from professionals who are genuinely concerned to help her have a vaginal birth if possible.

Obstetricians often quote statistics of uterine rupture in birth after a previous Caesarean. If you decide to go for a vaginal birth, say 'no' to induction and artificial stimulation of the uterus during labour. They increase the chances of uterine rupture. Even so, 370 Caesareans would need to be performed to prevent one uterine rupture without any symptoms.[165]

Remember that having an epidural makes it more likely that the baby will go to the nursery for diagnostic tests and interventions – because epidurals raise the baby's temperature to fever levels.[166]

159

A DOULA

There is evidence that continuous support is one of the best ways to have a positive experience and a natural birth.[167] A study of the relationship between nurses and women in labour in North America shows that unbroken emotional support is more important than having detailed information – more important than being held, touched and massaged, though you may want all of these, too.[168]

A birth companion, whether a doula or a midwife who gives good support, helps you tackle pain yourself so that you are less likely to need drugs. She responds to and understands how you are feeling, encourages and praises you, and uses touch to comfort, relieve pain and help you relax and work with your body instead of resisting the power of the contractions. This is not a matter of using techniques so much as the kind of person she is. That is vitally important in choosing a doula.

Studies in North America comparing obstetric nurses with doulas suggest that it is better if the birth companion is not employed by the hospital but selected by the woman, and that they should get to know each other before labour starts. Women who have this kind of care use fewer drugs for pain relief and are more likely to have a spontaneous vaginal birth.[169]

BIRTH AT HOME

Recent research into home birth shows that it is as safe as birth in hospital for a woman who does not have special risk factors, such as pre-eclampsia or a premature baby, and that there is less morbidity for both mother and baby. This was a methodologically vigorous study; it was prospective rather than retrospective, and all the women planned their births. They didn't happen to give birth outside hospital because they did not get there on time, for example, or because the birth was the outcome of a concealed pregnancy.[170]

The study covered 5,418 women in the US and Canada who sought home births attended by a professional midwife with whom they had a continuing relationship. Of these, 12.1 per cent were transferred to hospital during labour or after the birth. The mortality rate for the babies was low – 1.7 per thousand, comparable to low-risk births in hospitals. No mothers died. There were few obstetric interventions: only 4.7 per cent epidurals, 2.1 per cent episiotomies, 1.0 per cent forceps delivery, 6 per cent vacuum extractions and 3.7 per cent Caesareans. These rates were much lower than those for low-risk women who gave birth in hospital. Mothers and babies were less likely to be ill afterwards when birth took place at home rather than following a hospital birth, and 97 per cent of the mothers said that they were 'extremely' or 'very' satisfied', with 89.6 per cent saying they would choose the same midwife for another birth. These are impressive statistics and suggest that even in a country where home birth is not built in to the system, if there is good midwife care, it may be the best option for most women.

Anticipate resistance when you say that you would like a home birth. An NHS midwife tends to feel that she must cover herself, and the way she ensures this is to tell you to make an appointment with a consultant obstetrician. Senior obstetricians who approve of home birth are few and far between. The most positive response is likely to be something as mild as, 'I wouldn't recommend it.' But you may be threatened with death or brain damage to the baby and be told that you are irresponsible.

One woman, writing in *The Lancet* about her experience of seeking a home birth, told how, reading a book of mine, she realised that her anxieties surrounding birth had very little to do with physical pain, but everything to do with being dehumanised and gobbled up by a system that would process her as an object. So she went to her next antenatal appointment intent on organising herself a home birth.

She was prepared for resistance but imagined that it would take the form of a coherent counter-argument to her plan. 'Not me' said the obstetrician. She asked how she should start planning to have her baby at home. 'You have to ask the midwife – it will be her decision' the obstetrician said. She explained that she was not scheduled to see a midwife. 'Oh no, you will see a midwife', he said. 'You will be cared for by midwives when you come in during labour'.

'Isn't that a bit late to start discussing where the birth might take place? And, er, won't I be at home having the home birth – not in hospital?'

She opted out of the NHS and found an independent midwife. She had a very happy home birth.

LABOUR AT HOME AS LONG AS YOU CAN

If you are booked into hospital for the next birth, you may decide to stay at home as long as possible during labour. The earlier you are admitted, the greater the risk of unnecessary interventions.

161

A rule of thumb is to delay going in until contractions are coming every five minutes or less, and lasting 40 seconds or longer. This is a rough guide, because you will know if you have reached the point when you feel more secure in the place where you are going to give birth. Only you can judge that.

You may be told to come in if your membranes have ruptured, because the longer that labour lasts after they have gone the higher the risk of infection. But studies that lead to that conclusion are on women who have had vaginal examinations, and the longer you are in hospital the more numerous they are. Frequent examinations are linked to ascending infection.

Bear in mind how long it will take you to reach hospital. Do a few trial runs at different times of the day, rush hour included.

A BIRTH CENTRE

Birth centres are either free-standing or special midwifery-led parts of a hospital. They are low-tech units that give friendly, one-to-one care, and the midwives are committed to supporting normal childbirth.[171] At the Edgware Birth Centre, for example, low-risk women have 37 per cent fewer emergency Caesarean sections than in the neighbouring hospitals and 90 per cent fewer planned Caesareans. In the hospitals women have well over twice as many inductions and epidurals, almost four times the rate of episiotomy, and nearly four times as many instrumental deliveries.[172]

An American study of more than 12,000 women who had their babies in 84 birth centres showed that mortality and morbidity rates were the same as those for low-risk women in hospital, and that there were far fewer interventions.[173] This was true also for birth centres in Sweden,[174,175] Germany[176] and Australia.[177]

The trouble is that a woman is fortunate if she has a birth centre near her, and even if there is one, she may be screened out from going there because of risk factors. There is more about home birth and birth centres in my book, *Birth Your Way: Choosing Birth at Home or in a Birth Centre*, London, Dorling Kindersley, 2002.

USING A BIRTH POOL

Floating, lying and moving in water are not only ways of relieving pain. They may help birth unfold normally. Being in water tends to shorten labour and reduces interventions, the baby is more likely to be curled up in a good position for birth, it increases the chances of vaginal birth and it reduces the risk of episiotomy and perineal trauma.[178,179]

You can get out of a pool when you wish and you may like to labour in water but give birth on dry land. The water should be deep enough to cover your bump and come up to your breasts. The temperature should be comfortable, blood heat or just over, though you may get so hot in the second stage that it feels good to let it cool down a bit then. The baby's temperature in the uterus is always a little higher than the mother's, so you don't want to get so hot that the baby becomes feverish.

To make best use of a pool ensure that it is large enough for you to move freely and that you are not fixed in one position by a seat. The sides should be firm enough to support your weight if you want to lean against or over them. If you use a pool that anyone else has been in before it should be cleaned with a chlorine-releasing agent.

The baby's heart can be monitored with a hand-held Doppler designed to be used under water.

Drink plenty of water while you are in the pool because being in water increases the need for fluids. Leave the pool when you want to empty your bladder.

The baby should be born under the water, gently lifted out into the air after a minute or so, and rested on your tummy, at the level of your uterus, so that it can breathe easily, and you can welcome it.

Opiate drugs, such as pethidine, should not be used if you plan to give birth in water, since they can compromise the baby's breathing. Entonox (gas and oxygen) is fine. (For more information about water birth see Ethel Burns and Sheila Kitzinger, *Midwifery Guidelines for the Use of Water in Labour*, 2nd edition, 2005 (www.brookes.ac.uk/schools/shsc/research/publist.html! and http://sheilakitzinger.com).

If you plan to use a pool in hospital, ask first what their rules are about who may use it. In some hospitals no woman whose membranes have already ruptured is allowed in the pool. Sometimes women can use the pool only if they are five centimetres or more dilated. Many hospitals have only one pool, so if somebody else is in it, or if it has not yet been cleaned from previous use, you will not be able to use it. In some, only certain midwives attend water births, and if they do not happen to be on duty, a woman cannot use the pool. It may be possible for you to take in your own portable pool, so discuss this, too.

This is easier said than done. Though much lip service is paid to it, a shortage of midwives makes it difficult for midwifery managers to guarantee. The standard pattern is team midwifery, and these teams may consist of up to 16 midwives. It is much better for a midwife to have her own caseload and work with one or two other midwives whom the mother also gets to know. Research shows that women receiving one-to-one care rate it highly. They say that it helps communication and they get the information they need at the right time. A relationship with a midwife they already know stimulates self-confidence.

One-to-one midwifery is based on each midwife having her personal caseload instead of working on shifts. In *The New Midwifery: Science and Sensitivity in Practice*, Professor Lesley Page discusses ways of organising midwifery and points out that:

> *Practice has been influenced by a society in which a factory model has affected many forms of work and organisational life. Thus, the most common model of midwifery care over recent decades has been an assembly line approach with the woman progressing along the line at different points in her pregnancy.*[180]

Continuity of *carer* is the goal – not just continuity of care. That means:

> *Enabling midwives to organise their practice so that they may form a continuous working relationship with women in their care. It means enabling midwives to work with women through the whole of pregnancy, birth and the early weeks of newborn life, so that they may get to know each other and form a relationship that is based on trust between the two.*[181]

A midwife with a personal caseload is 'primary midwife' for 35 to 40 women a year, and second midwife for the same number. She usually works in a community-based group practice. This is quite different from a team system in which at least six midwives may share a caseload of 300 to 350 women. Though women are happier having at least some midwives whom they have seen before, team midwifery does not improve childbirth outcomes such as rates of induction, instrumental delivery and breastfeeding.[182] There are no randomised controlled trials of caseload midwifery, but studies show that when women can compare different models of care for different births they prefer to have a known midwife.[183] As well as reducing the Caesarean rate, personal care increases the chance of a normal labour and spontaneous vaginal birth.[184,185,186,187]

Some midwives like the factory system and don't want to have to manage their own time. But many are themselves happier with a caseload practice, more responsibility, and autonomy and flexibility in their work. It is not that the midwife tries to provide exclusive care on which a woman becomes dependent, but she escapes 'the fragmented system in which women moved between a confusing array of systems and carers, without the benefit of a continuing personal relationship', and being used as reserve workforce to be summoned when the hospital is busy.[188] Happier midwives make for happier mothers.

WHAT ABOUT A PRIVATE OBSTETRICIAN?

If you choose private care from a consultant obstetrician, you need to be sure that you are in harmony about what birth is, how you want it to be, and his or her role. We have seen already that in the UK women outside the NHS get more interventions of every kind, more drugs and more Caesarean sections. Unless you are sure that this is what you want, ask searching questions.

You might ask an obstetrician for the rate of normal births without interventions for women he or she has cared for in the last three years, for example, and if you can have the statistics for rates of induction of labour, instrumental births and Caesareans over that time.

Ina May Gaskin, a wise American midwife from the Farm in Tennessee advises, 'If any of your questions provoke resentment, sarcasm, hostility, scare tactics, or vague or patronising answers, keep shopping.'[189]

AN INDEPENDENT MIDWIFE?

Independent midwives are outside the NHS, though some – and this is an increasing practice – are hired by NHS Trusts to attend home births when there is a shortage of midwives to do this. Independent midwives also work in private birth centres. They have often left the NHS because they disapprove of the way women are treated and the dehumanisation of birth, and want to offer a better and more personal quality of care.

Find an independent midwife through The Independent Midwives Association (IMA), see 'Useful addresses' (pp. 169–73).

If you choose an independent midwife, discuss with her what will happen if you need to be transferred to hospital. Will she be accepted as your midwife and be able to continue caring for you in that hospital? Or will she not be welcome? Or only as an observer? Can discussion take place with the hospital authorities to make it easier if you need to be admitted?

Independent midwives are calling for one-to-one midwifery for all women having NHS care. Their One Mother, One Midwife campaign states that every woman should be able to choose her midwife and that the maternity services should be based on choice, information and partnership, as in the IMA's Community Midwifery Model. With this system there would be a national midwifery contract so that both midwives in the NHS and independent midwives could use NHS facilities to offer one-to-one care.[190]

LABOUR AND GIVING BIRTH IN ANY POSITION YOU CHOOSE

There is growing recognition that many women don't like lying with their legs strung up in stirrups, or flat on the back with just one or two flattened pillows for birth. Yet most still give birth lying down because it is expected of them – and they expect it of themselves. This is probably because in most hospitals the bed is positioned centrally in the birth room. The implicit message is: 'Get on it.'

Though midwives and doctors may prefer it because they think they have more control over the delivery, and that there is less blood if a woman is supine, there is no good reason for this.[191] When women can move around and be upright the rate of instrumental deliveries is reduced, the pushing stage is shorter, and they are less likely to need an episiotomy.[192]

In traditional cultures across the world woman usually give birth in upright or semi-upright positions.[193]

You don't need a special birth chair or stool. In fact, it is best to change position frequently and to use furniture and ledges in the room, a mat on the floor, perhaps a 'birth ball', foam wedge, pile of pillows, or another human body to support you so that you can rock your pelvis freely.

Sitting for a long time in one position can cause vulval congestion and swelling. It is better to switch between squatting, kneeling, half kneeling-half squatting, being on all fours, standing on bent knees, and forward leaning positions.

RESEARCH A BIRTH PLAN AND EXPLORE IT WITH
YOUR MIDWIFE

With a background of reading and research you will have a solid foundation on which to discuss a possible birth plan with your care-giver and develop it further. This is another reason why it is important to know your midwife. You are not just handing over a shopping list to whoever you happen to encounter when you are in labour. If you have not been able to build a relationship with your caregivers in pregnancy, they may not understand what you really want. They may get the idea that you are unrealistic, pig-headed and likely to be a 'difficult patient'.

Ask for time in which you can explore how to have a birth that is as undisturbed and gentle as possible.

A doctor mother, Sarah Buckley, whose own experience included an undisturbed persistent occipito-posterior delivery and a breech birth, puts it this way:

> *Anything that disturbs a labouring woman's sense of safety and privacy will disrupt the birth process. This definition covers most of modern obstetrics, which has created an entire industry around the observation and monitoring of pregnant and birthing women . . .*
>
> *On top of this is another obstetric layer diverted to correcting the 'dysfunctional labour' that such disruption is likely to produce. The resulting distortion of the process of birth – what we might call 'disturbed birth' – has come to be what women expect when they have a baby and perhaps, in a strange circu-larity, it works. Under this model women are almost certain to need the interventions that the medical model promotes, and to come away grateful to be saved no matter how difficult or trau-matic their experience.*[194]

167

Professor G. Kloosterman was a stalwart champion of mid-wifery and prevented the Netherlands from following the route to the aggressive active management of labour that proved enticing for obstetricians throughout the rest of the world. He summed up his approach when he wrote:

> *Spontaneous labour in a normal woman is an event marked by a number of processes so complicated and so perfectly attuned to each other that any interference will only detract from the*

optimal character. The only thing required from the bystanders is that they show respect for this awe-inspiring process by complying with the first rule of medicine – nil nocere (do no harm).'[195]

USEFUL ADDRESSES

Acupuncture
British Acupuncture Council
Tel: 020 8735 0400
www.acupuncture.org.uk

The baby
Attachment Parenting International
www.attachmentparenting.org

Birth
Active Birth Centre
Tel: 020 7281 6760
www.activebirthcentre.com

Association of Labor Assistants and Childbirth
    Educators (ALACE)
PO Box 390346, Cambridge, MA 02139
Tel: 617 441 2500
www.alace.org

Birth Crisis
Tel: 01865 300266
www.birthcrisis.sheilakitzinger.org

Childbirth.Org
www.childbirth.org

International Childbirth Education Association (ICEA)
PO Box 20048, Minneapolis, MN 54420
www.icea.org

Lamaze Institute for Normal Birth
2025 M Street NW, Suite 800, Washington, DC 20036-3309
www.lemaze.org/institute

Maternity Coalition Australia
www.maternity.coalition.org.au

National Childbirth Trust (NCT)
Tel: 0870 444 8707
www.nctpregnancyandbabycare.com

Trauma and Birth Stress (TABS)
www.tabs.org.nz

Birth Centres
Birth Centre Network (BCN-UK)
health.groups.yahoo.com/group/birthcentres/

Maternity Center Association
281 Park Avenue South, 5th floor, New York, NY 10010
www.maternitywise.org

National Association of Childbearing Centers (NACC)
3123 Gottschall Road, Perkiomenville, PA 18074
www.birthcenters.org

Breastfeeding
www.breastfeedingnetwork.org.uk
www.laleche.org.uk
www.laleche.com

Caesarean
International Cesarean Awareness Network (ICAN)
www.ican-online.org

Vaginal Birth after Caesarean
www.vbac.com

Counselling
Birth Trauma Association
PO Box 671, Ipswich IP1 9AT
www.birthtraumaassociation.org.uk

British Association for Counselling and Psychotherapy
Tel: 01788 550899
www.counselling.co.uk

British Association for Sexual and Relationship Therapy
Tel: 020 8543 2707
www.basrt.org.uk

Relate
Tel: 01788 573241
www.relate.org.uk

Doulas
Doula UK
Tel: 0871 433 3103
www.doula.org.uk

Doulas of North America (DONA)
PO Box 626, Jasper, IN 47457
www.dona.org

See also ALACE

Home birth
Home Birth Reference Site
www.homebirth.org.uk

Home Midwifery Association
www.homebirth.org.au

See also Birth Choice UK

Hynotherapy/midwife
HypnoBirthing
www.naturalchildbirth.co.uk

Natal Hypnotherapy
Tel: 01428 712615
www.natalhypnotherapy.com

Massage
Neuroendocrine responses to massage in late pregnancy, labour and post-natal:
theory and practice
www.childbirth-massage.co.uk

Maternity services
Association for Improvements in the Maternity Services (AIMS)
www.aims.org.uk

Association of Radical Midwives
www.radmid.demon.co.uk
Helpline Sarah Montagu, tel: 01865 248159

Birth Choice UK
www.birthchoiceuk.com

Independent Midwives' Association
Tel: 01483 821104
www.independentmidwives.org.uk

Royal College of Midwives
www.rcmnormalbirth.net

Mothers
Mothering Magazine
The magazine of natural family living
www.mothering.com

Mothers 35+
www.mothers35plus.co.uk

Pain
Midwives of Washington
Information and advice on giving sterile water injections to relieve back pain
www.midwivesofwa.org

Reflexology
Association of Reflexologists.
Tel. 0870 567 3320
www.aor.org.uk

Relaxation
Relaxation, meditation and reflexology
www.heartbeatwithin.co.uk

Research
Michel Odent's Primal Health Research
www.birthworks.org/primalhealth
www.michelodent.com

Midwives Information and Resource Service (MIDIRS)
www.midirs.org

Shiatsu
The Shiatsu Society
Tel: 0845 130 4566
www.shiatsu.org

TENS
Antenatal Results and Choices
Tel: 020 7631 0285
www.arc-uk.org

Yoga
Birthlight Trust
Tel: 01223 362288
www.birthlight.com

Kundalini yoga
Tel: 020 7708 2389
www.devotion.org.uk

NOTES

For an electronic version of these references, with relevant links, please go to www.sheilakitzinger.com/books/BCreferences.htm

CHAPTER 1 BIRTH SHOCK

1 J. Czarnocka and P. Slade, 'Prevalence and predictors of post-traumatic stress symptoms following childbirth', *Br. J. Clin. Psychol.*, 2000; 39: 35–51

2 D. K. Creedy, I. M. Shochnet and J. Horsfall, 'Childbirth and the development of acute trauma symptoms: incidence and contributing factors', *Birth*, 2000; 27: 104–11

3 D. Summerfield, 'The invention of post-traumatic stress disorder and the social usefulness of a psychiatric category', *British Medical Journal*, 2001; 322: 95–8

4 D. J. Murphy, C. Pope, J. Frost *et al.*, 'Women's views on the impact of operative delivery in the second stage of labour: qualitative interview study', *British Medical Journal*, 2003; 327: 1132–5

CHAPTER 2 BIRTH CONTRASTS

5 P. Simkin, 'Just another day in a woman's life? Part II: Nature and consistency of women's long-term memories in their first birth experiences', *Birth*, 1992; 19(2): 64–81

6 BBC Radio 4, 29 July 2005

7 K. O'Driscoll, D. Meagher and P. Boylam, *Active Management of Labour*, London, Mosby, 1993

8 O'Driscoll, Meagher and Boylam, *Active Management of Labour*: 44

9 O'Driscoll, Meagher and Boylam, *Active Management of Labour*: 79

10 MIDIRS, *Informed Choice, Leaflet for Professionals*, 2005. These leaflets are produced by the Midwives Information and Resource Service (MIDIRS) in collaboration with other various research groups. They are published by MIDIRS in Bristol. Web address for infochoice is www.infochoice.org.

11 M. Kirkham, H. Stapleton, P. Curtis *et al.*, 'Stereotyping as a professional defence mechanism', *British Journal of Midwifery*, 2002; 10(9): 549–52

12 Kirkham *et al.*, 'Stereotyping'

CHAPTER 3 INSTITUTIONAL POWER IN A HIGH-TECH BIRTH CULTURE

13 J. Donnison, *Midwives and Medical Men*, London, Heinemann, 1977

14 Dr J. A. Guinn, quoted in J. W. Leavitt, *Brought to Bed: Child-Bearing in America*, 1750–1950, New York, Oxford University Press, 1986

15 J. P. Fairbairn, 'The medical and psychological aspects of gynaecology', *Lancet II*, 1931: 999–1004, quoted in I. Loudon, 'Obstetric care, social class, and maternal mortality', *British Medical Journal*, 1986; 293: 606–8

16 J. Henry, *Causes and Preventions of Maternal Mortality*, London (publisher's name not available) 1929: 238, quoted in J. Carter and P. Duriez, *With Child: Birth Through the Ages*, Edinburgh, Mainstream Publishing, 1986

17 M. H. Jones, S. Bariks, H. N. Mangunhh *et. al.*, 'Do birth plans adversely affect the outcome of labour?', *British Journal of Midwifery* 1998; (1): 38–41

18 M. Moore and U. Hopper, 'Do birth plans empower women? Evaluation of hospital birth plans', *Birth*, 1995; 22(1): 99–103

19 J. Jolly, J. Walker and K. Bhabia, 'Subsequent obstetric performance related to primary mode of delivery', *British Journal of Obstetrics and Gynaecology*, 1999; 106(3): 227–32

20 D. Scully, *Men Who Control Women's Health*, Boston MA, Houghton Mifflin, 1980

21 *NHS Maternity Statistics, England: 2002–2003*, Government Statistical Service, London, 2004

22 M. Singata and J. E. Tranmer, 'Restricting oral fluid and food intake during labour', *The Cochrane Database of Systematic Reviews*, 2002, issue 4

23 Franca Pizzini, 'The woman patient in an obstetrical situation: communicative hierarchies in humour', paper presented at the Third International Interdisciplinary Congress of Women, held in Dubai, July 1987

24 S. B. Thacker, D. Stroup and M. Chang, 'Continuous electronic fetal heart rate monitoring for fetal assessment during labor', *The Cochrane Database of Systematic Reviews*, 2001, issue 2

25 *Listening to Mothers Survey*, Maternity Center Association, 2002, www.maternitywise.org/listeningtomothers/index.html

26 E. D. Hodnett, S. Gates, G. J. Hofmeyr *et al.*, 'Continuous support for women during childbirth', *The Cochrane Database of Systematic Reviews* 2003, issue 3

27 Thacker, Stroup and Chang, 'Continuous electronic fetal heart rate monitoring'

28 J. P. Nielson, 'Fetal electrocardiogram (ECG) for fetal monitoring during labour', *The Cochrane Database of Systematic Reviews*, 2003, issue 2

29 'Behind the mask', Editorial, *The Lancet 1*, 1981: 197–8
30 M. A. Hunter and D. Williams, 'Mask wearing in the labour ward', *Midwives Chronicle*, 1985; 12: 14
31 J. Roth, 'Ritual and magic in the control of contagion', *American Sociological Review*, 22, 1957
32 *NHS Maternity Statistics 2002–2003*, NHS, London: 2002/3
33 S. Kitzinger, *Some Women's Experiences of Episiotomy*, London: National Childbirth Trust, 1980

CHAPTER 4 MANAGING THE REPRODUCTIVE MACHINE

34 M. Gross, S. Drobnic and M. Kierse, 'Influence of fixed and time-dependent factors on duration of normal first stage of labor', *Birth*, 2005; 32(1): 27–33
35 K. Baker, 'Protecting the public – from me', *The Practising Midwife*, 2005; 8(8): 20–1
36 S. K. Cesario, 'Re-evaluation of Friedman's labor curve: a pilot study', *JOGNN: Journal of Obstetric, Gynecologic and Neonatal Nursing*, 2004; 33(6): 713–22
37 I. Chalmers, 'Evaluation of different approaches to obstetric care', *British Journal of Obstetrics and Gynaecology*, 1976; 83(12): 921–33
38 *NHS Maternity Statistics 2002–2003*, NHS, London: 2002/3
39 Chalmers, 'Evaluation of different approaches'
40 D. Richter, *The advantage of elective labour by a psychosomatic approach*, paper given at 5th International Congress of Psychosomatic Obstetrics and Gynaecology, Rome, 1977
41 S. Kitzinger, *Some Mothers' Experiences of Induced Labour*, 2nd edn, London, National Childbirth Trust, 1978
42 J. Selwyn-Crawford, 'Lumbar epidural analgesia for labour and delivery – a personal view', in R. Beard, M. Brudenell, P. Dunn *et al.*, *The Management of Labour*, London, Royal College of Obstetricians and Gynaecologists, 1975
43 P. Taipale and V. Hiilesmaa, 'Predicting delivery date by ultrasound and last menstrual period in early gestation', *Obstet. Gynecol.*, 2001; 97(2): 189–94
44 J. Rosser, 'Calculating the EDD: which is more accurate, scan or LMP?', *Practising Midwife* 2000; 3(3): 28–9, and T. F. Baskett and F. Naegele, 'Naegele's rule: a reappraisal', *British Journal of Obstetrics and Gynaecology (BJOG)*, 2000; 107(11): 1433–5
45 MIDIRS, *Informed Choice for Professionals: Prolonged Pregnancy*, January 2005, www.infochoice.org
46 World Health Organization Recommendations, Consensus Conference on Appropriate Technology, London: World Health Organization (WHO), 1985
47 B. P. Yawn, P. Wollan, K. McKeon *et al.*, *American Journal of Obstetrics and Gynecology*, 2001; 184(4): 611–19
48 Maternity Centre Association, *Listening to Mothers Survey*, London, 2002, www.maternitywise.org/listeningtomothers/index.html
49 Amnesty International, *Israel and the Occupied Territories – Conflict, Occupation and Patriarchy – Women Carry the Burden*, web.amnesty.org/library/index/engmde150162005

50 G. J. Hofmeyer and A. M. Gulmezoglu, 'Vaginal misoprostol for cervical ripening and induction of labour', Cochrane Review in *The Cochrane Library*, Issue 2, 2001, Oxford, Cochrane Update Software

51 Z. Alfrevic, 'Oral misoprostol for induction of labour', Cochrane Review in *The Cochrane Library*, issue 1, 2003, Oxford, Cochrane Update Software

52 J. M. Green and H. A. Baston, 'Feeling in control during labor: Concepts, correlates, and consequences', *Birth*, 2003; 30(4): 235–47

53 U. Waldenström, V. Berman and G. Vasell, 'The complexity of labor pain: experiences of 278 women', *J. Psychosom. Obstet. Gynecol.*, 1996; 11: 120–9

54 Royal College of Obstetricians and Gynaecologists, *Induction of Labour*, London, RCOG Press, 2001

55 I. Graham and C. Davis, 'Episiotomy: the unkindest cut', in C. Henderson and D. Bick, *Perineal Care: An International Issue*, Salisbury, Quay Books, 2005

56 A. Shorten and B. Shorten, 'Women's choice? 'The impact of private health insurance on episiotomy rates in Australian hospitals', *Midwifery,* 2000; 16(3): 204–12

57 C. M. Begley, 'Consumer demand for Caesarean sections in Brazil. Episiotomy rates may change after evidence based intervention', *Br. Med. J.*, 2002; 325(7359): 335

58 N. L. S. Howden, A. M. Weber and L. A. Meyn, 'Episiotomy use among residents and faculty compared with private practitioners', *Obstet. Gynecol.*, 2004; 103(1): 114–18

59 J. Goldberg, D. Holtz, T. Hyslop *et al.*, 'Has the use of routine episiotomy decreased? Examination of episiotomy rates from 1983 to 2000', *Obstet. Gynecol.*, 2002; 99(3): 395–400; A. M. Weber and L. Meyn, 'Episiotomy use in the United States 1979–1997', *Obstet. Gynecol.*, 2002; 100(6): 1177–82; and J. D. Weeks and L. J. Kozak, 'Trends in the use of episiotomy in the United States: 1980–1998', *Birth*, 2001; 28(3): 152–60

60 E. Burns, *Midwifery Guidelines on the Use of Water in Childbirth*, 2nd edn, Oxford, Oxford Brookes University, 2005

61 National Centre for Health Statistics, London, Routledge, 2003

62 E. Declercq, F. Menacker and M. MacDorman, 'Rise in "no indicated risk" primary caesareans in the United States, 1991–2001: cross sectional analysis', *British Medical Journal*, doi:10.1136/bmj.38279.705336.0B, November 2004

63 B. P. Perkins, *The Medical Delivery Business: Health Reform, Childbirth and the Economic Order*, New Jersey: Rutgers University Press, 2004

64 S. Hodges and H. Goer, 'Effects of hospital economics on maternity care', *Citizens for Midwifery News*, Spring/Summer 2004

65 Perkins, *The Medical Delivery Business*

66 Hodges and Goer, 'Effects of hospital economics'

67 *Care of Women in US Hospitals*, 2000, HCUP Fact Book No. 3

68 M. Hall, 'Caesarean section', in G. Lewis (ed.), *Why Mothers Die 1997–1999: the Fifth Report of the Confidential Enquiries into Maternal Deaths in the United Kingdom*, London, RCOG Press, 2001: 317–22

69 G. Lewis (ed.) *Why Mothers Die 1997–1999: the Fifth Report of the Confidential Enquiries into Maternal Deaths in the United Kingdom*, London, RCOG Press, 2001

70 L. J. Burrows, L. A. Meyn and A. M. Weber, 'Maternal morbidity associated with vaginal versus Cesarean delivery', *Obstet. Gynecol.*, 2004; 103(5): 907–12

71 T. Singh, C. W. Justin and R. K. Haloob, 'An audit on trends of vaginal delivery after one previous Caesarean section', *Obstet. Gynaecol.*, 2004; 24(2): 135–8

72 H. Aslan, E. Unlu, M. Agor *et al.*, 'Uterine rupture associated with misoprostol labor induction in women with previous Cesarean delivery', *Eur. J. Obstet. Gynecol. Reprod. Biol.*, 2004; 113(1): 45–8

73 American College of Obstetricians and Gynecologists, 'Induction of labor for vaginal birth after Cesarean delivery', *Obstet. Gynecol.*, 2002; 99(4): 679–80

74 J. J. Morrison, J. M. Rennie and P. J. Milton, 'Neonatal respiratory morbidity and mode of delivery at term: Influence of timing of elective Caesarean section', *Br. J. Obstet. Gynaecol.*, 1995; 102(2): 101–6

75 V. Zanardo, A. K. Simbi, M. Franzoi *et al*, 'Neonatal respiratory morbidity risk and mode of delivery at term: influence of timing of elective Caesarean delivery', *Acta Paediatr.*, 2004; 93(5): 643–47

76 D. J. Annibale, T. C. Hulsey, C. L. Wagner *et al.*, 'Comparative neonatal morbidity of abdominal and vaginal deliveries after uncomplicated pregnancies', *Arch Pediatrics and Adolescent Med.*, 1995; 149(8): 862–7

77 M. Enkin, M. J. N. C. Keirse, J. Neilson *et al.*, *A guide to effective care in pregnancy and childbirth*, Oxford: Oxford University Press, 2000

78 J. Grinstead and W. A. Grobman, 'Induction of labor after one prior Cesarean: predictors of vaginal delivery', *Obstet. Gynecol.*, 2004; 103(3): 534–8

79 A. O. Odibo and G. A. Macones, 'Current concepts regarding vaginal birth after Cesarean delivery', *Current Opinion Obstet. Gynecol.*, 2003; 15(6): 479–82

179

CHAPTER 5 SEXUAL ABUSE AND BIRTH

80 J. Kitzinger, 'Recalling the pain', *Nursing Times,* 1990; 86(3): 38–40

81 J. Kitzinger, 'Counteracting, not re-enacting, the violation of women's bodies: the challenge for perinatal care-givers', *Birth,* 1992; 19(4): 119–220

82 P. Simkin, 'Memories that really matter', *Childbirth Instructor Magazine,* 1994; 39: 20–3

83 S. Fraser, *My Father's House: A Memoir of Incest and Healing*, New York: Harper & Row, 1990

84 M. Lesnik-Oberstein, 'Iatrogenic rape of a fourteen-year-old girl: a note', *Child Abuse and Neglect,* 1982; 6: 103–4

85 L. Armstrong, *Kiss Daddy Goodnight*, New York, Pocket Books, 1987

86 E. Burns and S. Kitzinger, *Midwifery Guidelines for the Use of Water in Labour*, Oxford, Oxford Brookes University, 2005

87 Anon, *Parents Magazine*, Australia, August/September, 1993

88 C. Burke Draucker, *Counseling Survivors of Childhood Sexual Abuse*, Newbury Park CA, Sage Publications, 1992

89 P. Simkin and P. Klaus, *When Survivors Give Birth; Understanding and Healing the Effects of Early Sexual Abuse on Childbearing Women*, Seattle WA, Classic Day Publishing, 2004

CHAPTER 6 FLASHBACKS, PANIC ATTACKS AND NIGHTMARES

90 American Psychiatric Association DSM–IV-TR, *Diagnostic and Statistical Manual of Mental Disorders*, 4th edn, text revision, Washington DC, 2000

91 G. Mezey and I. Robbins, 'Usefulness and validity of post-traumatic stress disorder as a psychiatric category', *British Medical Journal*, 2001; 323: 561–3

92 National Institute of Mental Health Association, *Post Traumatic Stress Disorder*, www.nmha.org

CHAPTER 7 PAIN

93 E. D. Hodnett, 'Pain and women's satisfaction with the experience of childbirth: a systematic review', *Am. J. Obstet. Gynecol.*, 2002; 186(5) (suppl.): S160–72

94 M. M. Gross, H. Hecker and M. J. N. C. Keirse, 'An evaluation of pain and 'fitness' during labor and its acceptability to women', *Birth*, 2005; 32(2): 122–8

95 MIDIRS, 'Non-epidural strategies for pain relief during labour', *MIDIRS Midwifery Digest*, January 2005

96 J. W. Whitridge, *Obstetrics: A Textbook for the Use of Students and Practitioners*, New York and London, D. Appleton and Company, 1930.

97 J. Wolf, 'Mighty glad to gasp in the gas: perceptions of pain and the traditional timing of obstetric anaesthesia', *Health: an interdisciplinary journal for the social study of health, illness and medicine*, London: Sage, 2002; 6(3): 365–87

98 J. M. Green and H. A. Baston, 'Feeling in control during labor: concepts, correlates, and consequences', *Birth*, 2003; 30(4): 235–47.

99 U. Waldenström, 'Women's memory of childbirth at two months and one year after the birth', *Birth*, 2003; 30(4): 248–54

100 G. Chamberlain, A. S. Wraight and P. Steer (eds), *Pain and its Relief in Childbirth: the Results of a National Survey Conducted by the National Birthday Trust*, Edinburgh, Churchill Livingstone, 1993

101 J. E. Mattingly, J. D'Alessio and J. Ramanathan, 'Effects of obstetric analgesics and anaesthetics on the neonate: a review', *Pediatr. Drugs*, 2003; 5(9): 615–27

102 L. Bricker and T. Lavender, 'Parenteral opioids for labor pain relief: a systematic review', *Am. J. Obstet. Gynecol.*, 2002; 186(5) (suppl.): S94–109

103 L. Righard and M. O. Alade, 'Effect of delivery room routines on success of first breast-feed', *Lancet*, 1990; 336(8723): 1105–7

104 A. Ransjö-Arvidson, A. Matthiesen, G. Lilja *et al.*, 'Maternal analgesia during labor disturbs newborn behavior: effects on breastfeeding, temperature, and crying', *Birth*, 2001; 28(1): 5–12

105 E. Lieberman and C. O'Donoghue, 'Unintended effects of epidural analgesia during labor: a systematic review', *Am. J. Obstet. Gynecol.*, 2002; 186: S31–68

106 *NHS Maternity Statistics* 2002–2003

107 D. M. Levy, 'Analgesia and anaesthesia', in D. T. Y. Liu (ed.), *Labour Ward Manual*, 3rd edn, Edinburgh, Churchill Livingstone, 2003: 57–70

108 Mattingly, D'Alessio and Ramanathan, 'Effects of obstetric analgesics'

109 J. B. Hill, J. M. Alexander, S. K. Sharma *et al.*, 'A comparison of the effects of epidural and meperidine analgesia during labor on fetal heart rate', *Obstet. Gynecol.*, 2003; 102(2): 333–7

110 Lieberman and O'Donoghue, 'Unintended effects of epidural analgesia'

111 A. Thallon and A. Shennan, 'Epidural and spinal analgesia and labour', *Curr. Opin. Obstet. Gynecol.*, 2001; 13(6): 583–7

112 C. J. Howell, T. Dean, L. Lucking *et al.*, 'Randomised study of long term outcome after epidural versus non-epidural analgesia during labour', *British Medical Journal*, 2002; 325: 357–9

113 S. K. Sharma, J. M. Alexander, G. Messick *et al.*, 'Cesarean delivery: a randomised trial of epidural analgesia versus intravenous meperidine analgesia during labor in nulliparous women', *Anesthesiology*, 2002; 96(3): 546–51

114 J. E. Dickinson, M. J. Paech, S. J. McDonald *et al.*, 'The impact of intrapartum analgesia on labour and delivery outcomes in nulliparous women', *Aust. NZ J. Obstet. Gynaecol.*, 2002; 42: 59–66

115 Comparative Obstetric Mobile Epidural Trial (COMET) Study Group UK, 'Effects of low-dose mobile versus traditional epidural techniques on mode of delivery: a randomised controlled trial', *Lancet*, 2001; 358(9275): 19–23

116 J. G. Thornton and G. Capogna, 'Commentary: Reducing likelihood of instrumental delivery with epidural anaesthesia', *Lancet*, 2001; 358 (9275): 2

117 M. Fitzpatrick, R. Harkin and K. McQuillan, 'A randomised clinical trial comparing the effects of delayed versus immediate pushing with epidural analgesia on mode of delivery and faecal continence', *MIDIRS Midwifery Digest*, September 2003; 13(2): 215–16

118 L. Ching-Chung, C. Shuenn-Dhy, T. Ling-Hong *et al.*, 'Postpartum urinary retention: assessment of contributing factors and long-term clinical impact', *Aust. NZ J. Obstet. Gynaecol.*, 2002; 42: 365–8

119 M. Fitzpatrick, R. Harkin, K. McQuillan *et al.*, 'A randomised clinical trial comparing the effects of delayed versus immediate pushing with epidural analgesia on mode of delivery and faecal continence', *BJOG*, 2002; 109: 1359–65

120 U. Waldenström, I. Hildingsson, C. Rubertsson *et al.*, 'A negative birth experience: prevalence and risk factors in a national sample', *Birth*, 2004; 31(1); 17–27

CHAPTER 8 OTHER WAYS OF HANDLING PAIN

121 E. D. Hodnett, S. Gates, G. J. Hofmeyr *et al.*, 'Continuous support for women during childbirth', *The Cochrane Database of Systematic Reviews*, 2003, issue 3

122 M. Odent, 'Comments on "Parturition pain treated by intracutaneous injections of sterile water", by L. Ader, B. Handsson, G. Wallin, *Pain*, 41 (1990) 133–138)', *Pain*, 1991, 45: 220

123 P. Simkin and M. O'Hara, 'Nonpharmacologic relief of pain during labor: systematic reviews of five methods', *Can. Fam. Physician*, 1998; 44: 2391–2

124 L. Martensson and G. Wallin, 'Labour pain treated with cutaneous injections of sterile water: a randomised controlled trial', *Br. J. Obstet. Gynaecol.*, 1999; 106(7): 633–7

125 E. Skilnand, D. Fossen and E. Heiburg, 'Acupuncture in the management of pain in labor', *Acta Obstet. Gynecol. Scand.*, 2002; 81(10): 943–8

126 B. Nesheim, R. Kinge, B. Berg *et al.*, 'Acupuncture during labor can reduce the use of meperidine: a controlled clinical study', *Clin. J. Pain*, 2003; 9(3): 187–91

127 S. T. Brown, C. Douglas and L. P. Flood, 'Women's evaluation of intrapartum nonpharmacological pain relief methods used during labor', *J. Perinat. Educ.*, 2001; 10(3): 1–8

128 A. Ramnero, U. Hanson and M. Kihlgren, 'Acupuncture treatment during labour – a randomized controlled trial', *BJOG*, 2002; 109(6): 637–44

129 S. Yates, *Shiatsu for Midwives*, Oxford, Books for Midwives, 2003

130 S. Yates, 'Shiatsu and acupressure in practice', *MIDIRS Midwifery Digest*, 2005; 15(1): S35-S38

131 S. Emzer, *Reflexology: A Tool for Midwives*, The Association of Reflexologists, www.aor.org.uk

132 W. Conkling, *Hypnosis for a Joyful Pregnancy and Pain-Free Labor and Delivery*, New York, Lynn Sonberg, St Martin's Griffin, 2002

133 Conkling, *Hypnosis for a Joyful Pregnancy*

134 S. Kitzinger, *The New Experience of Childbirth*, London, Orion, 2004

135 L. Slater, *Love Works Like This: Travels Through a Pregnant Year*, London, Bloomsbury, 2003

136 E. R. Cluett, V. C. Nikodem, R. E. McCandlish *et al.*, 'Immersion in water in pregnancy, labour and birth', *The Cochrane Database of Systematic Reviews*, 2004, issue I

137 V. Geissbuhler and J. Eberhard, 'Waterbirths: a comparative study', *Fetal Diagn. Ther.*, 2000; 15(5): 291–300

138 V. Geissbuhler, S. Stein and J. Eberhard, 'Waterbirths compared with landbirths: an observational study of nine years', *J. Perinat. Med.*, 2004; 32(4): 308–14

139 A. Thoni and L. Moroder, 'Waterbirth: a safe and natural delivery method: experience after 1355 waterbirths in Italy', *Midwifery Today*, 2004; 70: 44–8

140 E. Burns and S. Kitzinger, *Midwifery Guidelines for Use of Water in Labour*, 2nd edn, Oxford, Oxford Brookes University, 2005

CHAPTER 9 'IF ONLY I HADN'T'

141 D. Pollock, *Telling Bodies: Performing Birth*, New York, Columbia University Press, 1999

142 Anon, 'Nathaniel's birth', *Interaction*: National Association of Childbirth Educators Incorporated, Australia, 2003; 21(3): 11–12

143 Letter in *Birthing,* Winter 2004: 43–4

CHAPTER 10 THE BABY

144 L. Slater, *Love Works Like This: Travels Through a Pregnant Year*, London, Bloomsbury, 2004: 121–2

145 Slater, *Love Works Like This*: 138

CHAPTER 11 THE PARTNER

146 Colin Dexter, *The Daughters of Cain*, London, Pan Books, 1995: 9

147 I. D. Graham, *Episiotomy: Challenging Obstetric Interventions*, Oxford, Blackwell Science, 1997:113–14

148 Graham, *Episiotomy*:116–17

149 Z. Nelson, 'The knives are out', *The Independent on Sunday*, Sunday Review, 3 July 2005

150 E. Samuelsson, L. Ladfors, UB. Wennerholm *et al.*, 'Anal sphincter tears: prospective study of obstetric risk factors', *BJOG,* 2000; 107(7): 926–31

151 A. Williams, T. Lavender, D. Richmond *et al.*, 'Women's experiences after a third degree obstetric anal sphincter tear: a qualitative study', *Birth*, 2005: 32(2): 129–36

CHAPTER 12 MOVING FORWARD

152 P. Simkin, 'Just another day in a woman's life? Part II: Nature and consistency of women's long-term memories of their first birth experiences', *Birth*, 1992; 19(2): 64–81

153 V. Taylor, *Rock-a-By Baby*, New York and London, Routledge, 1996

154 J. W. Leavitt, *Brought to Bed: Childbearing in America 1750–1950*, New York, Oxford University Press, 1986: 14

155 V. Clayton, S. Fishcein and J. Weckl, *Fearless Pregnancy: Wisdom and Reassurance from a Doctor, a Midwife, and a Mom*, Gloucester MA, Fairwinds Press, 2004: 204–5

156 www.tokophobia.com

157 M. Buber, *I and Thou* (trans. Ronald Gregor Smith), London, T. & T. Clark, 1937

158 D. Summerfield, 'Coping with the aftermath of trauma', letter, *British Medical Journal*, 2005; 331(7507): 50

159 *Poems of William Wordsworth*, London: Routledge

CHAPTER 13 PREGNANT AGAIN

160 S. Bewley and J. Cockburn, 'Should doctors perform Caesareans for "informed choice" alone?' in M. Kirkham, *Informed Choice in Maternity Care,* New York, Palgrave Macmillan, 2004

161 F. Ingelfinger, 'Arrogance', *New Eng. J. Med.,* 1980; 303: 1507–11 in Bewley and Cockburn, 'Should doctors perform Caesareans'

162 Bewley and Cockburn, 'Should doctors perform Caesareans'

163 T. Allen, R. Callender, S. Radley *et al.*, 'Multiple post-Caesarean pelvic floor symptoms can occur in young primiparae', paper presented at Marcé Society International Biennial Scientific Meeting, Oxford, September 2004

164 M. Enkin, M. J. N. C. Keirse, James Neilson *et al.*, *A Guide to Effective Care in Pregnancy and Childbirth*, Oxford, Oxford University Press, 2000

165 J. M. Guise, M. S. McDonagh, P. Osterweil *et al.*, 'Systematic review of the incidences and consequences of uterine rupture in women with previous Caesarean section', *British Medical Journal,* 2004; 329(7456): 19–23

166 R. Fisler, A. Cohen, S. Ringer *et al.*, 'Neonatal outcome after trial of labor compared with elective repeat cesarean section', *Birth*, 2003; 30(2): 83–8

167 E. D. Hodnett, S. Gates, G. J. Hofmeyr *et al.*, 'Continuous support for women during childbirth', *The Cochrane Database of Systematic Reviews*, 2003, issue 3

168 C. A. Corbett and L. C. Callister, 'Nursing support during labor', *Clin. Nurs. Res.*, 2000; 9: 70–83

169 Hodnett, Gates and Hofmeyr, 'Continuous support for women'

170 K. C. Johnson and B. Davis, 'Outcomes of planned home births with certified professional midwives: large prospective study in North America', *British Medical Journal*, 2005; 330: 1416

171 J. Rosser, 'Birth centres – the key to modernising the maternity services', *MIDIRS Midwifery Digest*, 2001; 11(2): S22-S26

172 D. Saunders, M. Boulton, J. Chapple *et al.*, *Evaluation of the Edgware Birth Centre,* Harrow, Northwick Park Hospital, North Thames Perinatal Public Health, 2000

173 J. P. Rooks, N. L. Weatherby and E. K. M. Ernst, 'The National Birth Centre Study, Part 11, Intrapartum and immediate postpartum and neonatal care', *Journal of Nurse Midwifery*, 1992; 37(5): 301–30

174 U. Waldenström, C. A. Nilsson and B. Winbladh, 'The Stockholm Birth Centre Trial: maternal and infant outcomes', *British Journal of Obstetrics and Gynaecology,* 1997; 104(4): 410–18

175 U. Waldenström and C. A. Nilsson, 'A randomized controlled study of birth center care versus standard maternity care: effects on women's health', *Birth*, 1997; 24(1): 17–26

176 M. David, H. K. Von Schwarzenfeld, J. A. S. Dimer *et al.*, 'Perinatal outcome in hospital and birth center obstetric care', *International Journal of Gynecology and Obstetrics,* 1999; 65(2): 149–56

177 A. Whelan, *Centering Birth: A Prospective Cohort Study of Birth Centers and Labour Wards*, Sydney: University of Sydney, Dept. of Public Health, 1994

178 E. Burns, 'Waterbirth', *MIDIRS Midwifery Digest*, 11:3(2): S10-S12

179 E. Burns and S. Kitzinger, *Midwifery Guidelines for the Use of Water in Labour*, 2nd edn, Oxford, Oxford Brookes University, 2005

180 C. McCourt, T. Stephens, J. Sandall *et al.*, 'Working with women: developing continuity of carer in practice', in L. A. Page, *The New Midwifery, Science and Sensitivity in Practice*, London, Churchill Livingstone, 2000

181 McCourt, Stephens and Sandall, 'Working with women'

182 E. D. Hodnett, 'Continuity of caregivers for care during pregnancy and childbirth, Cochrane Review', in *The Cochrane Library*, issue 4, Chichester, John Wiley & Sons, 2003, March 1999

183 C. McCourt and A. Pearce, 'Does continuity of carer matter to women in minority ethnic groups?', *Midwifery*, 2000; 16(2): 145–54

184 Y. Benjamin, D. Walsh and N. Taub, 'A comparison of partnership case-load midwifery care with conventional team midwifery care: labour and birth outcomes', *Midwifery*, 2001; 17: 234–40

185 The North Staffordshire Changing Childbirth Research Team, 'A randomised study of midwifery caseload and traditional "shared care"', *Midwifery*, 2000; 16: 295–302

186 J. Sandall, J. Davies and C. Warwick, *Evaluation of the Albany Midwifery Practice Final Report, Nightingale School of Nursing and Midwifery*, London, King's College, 2001

187 L. Page, S. Beake, A. Vail *et al.*, 'Clinical outcomes of one-to-one midwifery practice', *British Journal of Midwifery*, 2001; 9(11): 700–6

188 L. Page and R. McCandlish, *The New Midwifery*, London, Churchill Livingstone, 2006: 125

189 I. M. Gaskin, *Ina May's Guide for Childbirth*, New York, Bantam, 2003: 310

190 www.onemotheronemidwife.org.uk

191 E. D. Hodnett, 'Home-like versus conventional institutional settings for birth', *The Cochrane Database of Systematic reviews*, 2001, issue 4

192 Hodnett, Gates and Hofmeyr, 'Continuous support for women'

193 S. Kitzinger, *Rediscovering Birth*, London, Little Brown, 2000

194 S. Buckley, *Gentle Birth, Gentle Mothering*, Birthinternational.com, 2006: 74

195 G. Kloosterman, 'The universal aspects of childbirth: Human birth as a socio-psychosomatic paradigm', *J. Psychosom. Obstet. Gynaecol.*, 1982; 1(1): 35–41

INDEX

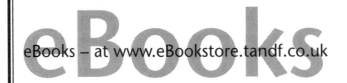